The Ninja Diet by David Watson.

Other Books from the Author:

I0776759

The ABC's of Rifle Shooting
The Mosin Nagant Performance Tuning Manual
The Lee Enfield Performance Tuning Manual
The Mauser M98 Performance Tuning Manual
The K31 Schmidt Rubin Performance Tuning Manual
The M38 Carcarno Performance Tuning Manual
The T38 Arisaka Performance Tuning Manual

The M38 Swedish Mauser Performance Tuning Manual
The P14 and M1917 Performance Tuning Manual
The M1903 Springfield Performance Tuning Manual

Marksmanship Masterclass

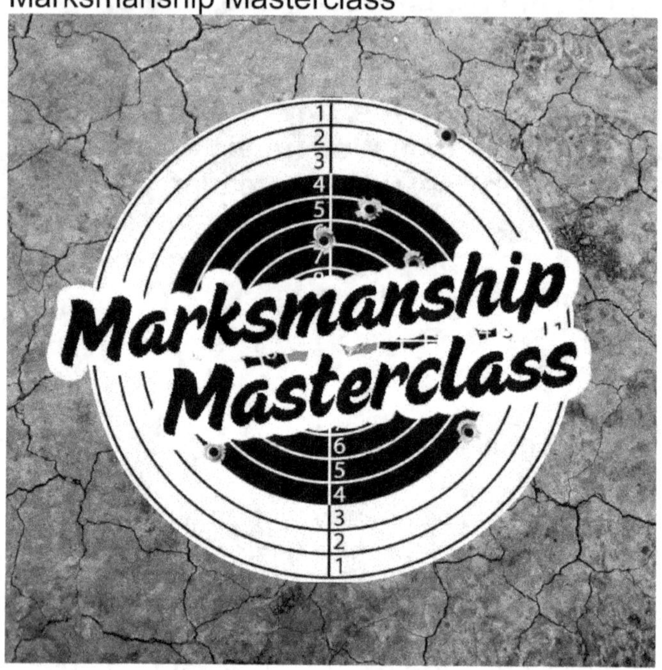

Books may be purchased by contacting the publisher and author at:
David Watson Gunsmith and Author
http://islandaccuracy.wixsite.com/abc-rifle-shooting

Library of Congress Catalog Number: xxx
ISBN: 9781982911324

First Edition
Printed in U.S.A

Contents

Disclaimer

The techniques and procedures in this book are given for academic study only. It is not the intention of the author, publisher, and distributors of this book to encourage the readers to perform any techniques or procedures herein. Attempting to do so can result in severe injury or death. The author, publisher, and distributors disclaim any liability for any loss, claim, damage or injury of any type, howeverso arising, whether in tort (including without limitation negligence), contract, statute equity or otherwise, that any reader, bystander or user of information contained within this book suffers as a result of or in connection with the use, misuse, or otherwise of the information contained herein.

Introduction

The *Ninja* are perhaps the most idealised and least understood warriors of all time. Their reputation for skill, daring and ability are unrivaled in the annals of history, and their methods, techniques and ways are shrouded in mystery and intrigue. What is known is that the Ninja were very much spiritual and agrarian in their existences and this is the root of their strengths that we can learn from.

The Ninja Diet is a plan designed to develop physical and mental fortitude, strength and toughness and is based on sensible and balanced eating coupled with lessons, legends and techniques from the past.

The Ninja Diet is intended to supplement into a person's regular eating patterns and in this way the Ninja Diet can play a role in developing ourselves without becoming a burden or a chore. In fact after several weeks the reader will not only be reaping the rewards of their efforts but will also being doing so effortlessly.

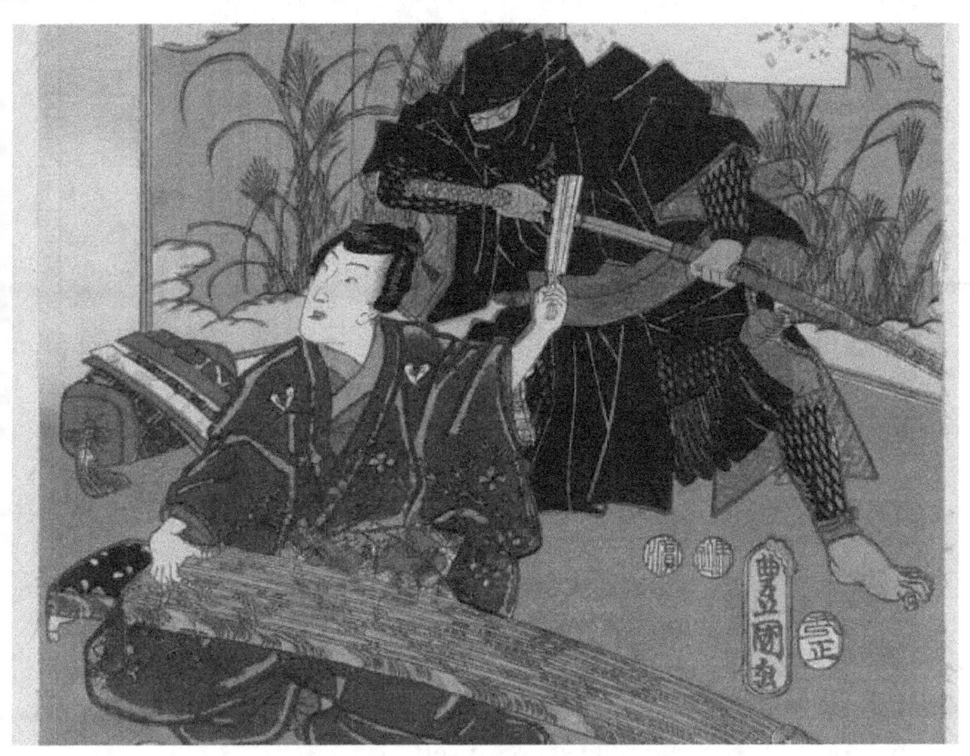

An 1852 woodblock depicting the contemporised view of the Ninja.

How to use this book

This book is not a dieting book for the body but a cleansing book for the mind. This book is a recipe for a new philosophy for the modern age, based on the lessons of the past.

Central to the feudal warrior traditions of Japan is the concept of '*Mu*' or '*Mushin*' – to be mindless or without mind. This is regularly translated poorly into 'not thinking' and this is far from the case. '*Mushin*' is better translated as 'mindfulness' and embodies the concept of being aware and connected to the moment, without being emotionally controlled by it.

The lessons within this book focus on a sensory diet to regulate and ground the mind, *Haiku* or Japanese poems to bring about internalisation and contemplation, and legends to stimulate the imagination and redevelop the sense of self.

The purpose of this book is not to have a 'two week fat burning blitz' or be the new 'six minute ab's'. The purpose of this book is to teach us how to learn about ourselves through food, history and culture, and develop a 'lean-ness' of body and mind, and not just become 'thin'.

The reader will note the prevalence of the number '9' within this book. There are nine recipes, nine *Kuji-In*, nine legends and so on. In the Japanese language, the word 'nine' can be pronounced as either '*Kyu*' or '*Ku*', with the former being considered a lucky number that sounds like the word for 'relief' and the latter being an unlucky number and sounding like the word for 'torture'. This recognises that change is difficult and painful however lasting change brings lasting gifts beyond face value.

The way of change is the way of persistence, and persistence is built on courage, belief and sense of new self, and so this book is a never ending circle. In fact it is an uplifting spiral, and if the reader takes a single step and considers it the journey, the journey will bring itself to the reader, and the reader will attain a sense of '*Mushin*'.

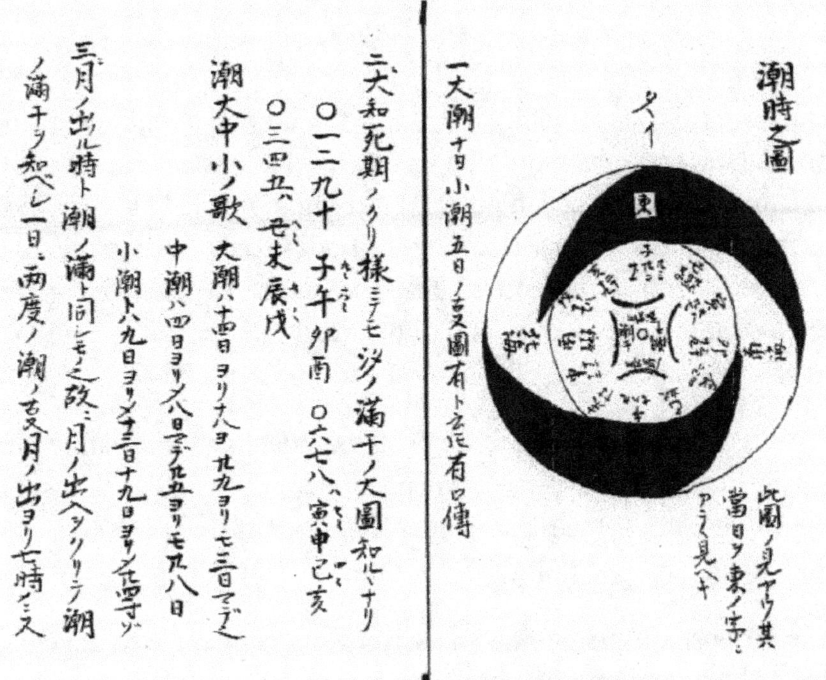

A page from the Bansenshukai written by Fujibayashi Sabuji circa 1676 detailing some of the more spiritual aspects of the Ninja.

The Diet

The term 'diet' is typically only used to describe a regimen of food consumption. However, the word diet can be used to describe anything that is consumed. For instance, a person listening to music has a musical diet of preferred song's, a person who reads books has a reading diet of preferred authors. In fact, our entire being and human experience can be considered a diet, and we need to think holistically like this if we are to adapt and change to better ourselves.

When considered this way, we need to understand that eating is only one part, likewise most people consider exercise to be the next step, but few go beyond this – the result is that followers of these practices become one thing, and one thing only – 'thin'.

The purpose of this book is to assist every day people to develop a 'lean-ness' of body and mind. To develop a sense of inner calm and physical strength, along with an indefatigable psychology and spirit.

The intention of this book is that the reader incorporates one of the nine lessons into their lives every day, and follows one of the nine lessons, every day. The reader, practice and perform one *Kuji-In* every day. The reader contemplate and internalise one *Haiku* every day. The reader consider one legend every day. The reader prepare and eat one meal from this book additional to their regular eating patterns every day.

The sharp eyed reader will notice a natural emphasis on both Paleo and Ketogenic diets within the Japanese diet, however this maintains a semblance of balance. It needs to be recognised that although the Paleo and Ketogenic diets focus on exclusive eating patterns, the historical record suggests that both diets in their historical use are survival diets, and if starchy vegetables or grains were available on any given day, they would be consumed, although perhaps not in agricultural quantities. The traditional Japanese diet focuses heavily on this sense of balance, and while there is an amount of rice, beans and wheat products, the rice is brown, the wheat is heavily portion controlled and the beans are fermented.

The first three recipes in this book are recognised as specific foods the *Ninja* used for specific purposes, and can be considered as power or energy snacks, specifically. They are not intended to be eaten every day. The remaining recipes focus on the common food eaten by the common folk of the era, and speak to the frugal agrarian lives that were lead by the people of the time. These recipes can be cooked and eaten every day. It should be noted that classes of ingredients are mentioned not specific ingredients – this is important as it requires the reader to adapt, change and remain flexible, much in the way *Ninja* did.

Hand in hand with food intake is Hydration and salt balance. Hydration is a simple term that describes a complex set of bio-chemical reactions in the body. More specifically, hydration deals with maintaining the correct concentration of water and salt within the body. As a rule of thumb the average person in a rested state, in temperate conditions, requires a minimum of 1Lt of water per day. Where a person is undergoing normal daily activities with some exertion, this figure can easy rise to 3–5Lts per day. Under extreme conditions, 1lt per hour may be required to maintain water balance. Of course, due to the constraints of modern life, few people actually hydrate appropriately and to the correct level. The effects of dehydration initially include, lethargy, lack of concentration and headaches, leading to blurred vision and difficulty with simple arithmetic.

It is important to note that a feeling of 'thirst' is reactionary response to dehydration. If we feel 'thirsty', we are already suffering the initial effects of dehydration. The best way to avoid dehydration is to regularly sip fresh water. It is important not to gulp water. Gulping tends to waste water as the body cannot absorb the water fast enough, and further, an overload of water in the stomach causes discomfort such as 'stitches'.

When a person perspires, not only are they loosing moisture from the body, they are also loosing salts. The effects of salt imbalance are far more difficult to detect as they mirror the effects of dehydration, except for a feeling of thirst. The key symptoms of mild salt imbalance separate to those of dehydration include muscle cramping, a need to urinate almost directly after consuming water and a general weakness of the body. Again, the best way to avoid salt imbalance is pre-emptive salt balance monitoring and manipulation. Likewise with water consumption, more is not better. Salt absorption is best achieved with small amounts of salt, dissolved in large amounts of water, then regularly sipped. A concentration of no more than 1/4 metric teaspoon of good quality sea salt per litre of fresh water is required. The water should taste barely tainted by the salt and should be easy to consume. It should be noted that there are many electrolyte solutions commercially available that contain the relevant salts, along with sugars and flavours, in both a liquid and powder form. These products tend to stress the body by placing many complex molecules into the stomach, requiring the body's organs to work hard to digest and absorb the necessary salts and sugars and as such, can lead to an increased heart rate and breathing which is not desirable.

It also needs to be recognised that art and science of maintaining a healthy body and mind requires that the body be exercised. General fitness in any discipline doesn't necessarily require us to be a fitness guru or work out several times a week at the gym. Of course, a higher level of physical fitness can only do you good; it does tend to offer diminishing returns for effort. So, what does all this mean for us, and what can we learn from the traditional Japanese diet, and the diet of the *Ninja*?

When we talk about physical fitness, we are talking about cardio-vascular fitness and pulmonary fitness, or in essence, how efficiently the heart and lungs work. Fortunately for us, heart and lung fitness pretty well go hand in hand, and the same exercise will address both areas. Another point of interest is weight versus height, and flexibility. The 'Body Mass

Index' (BMI) is a useful but simple tool for comparing height and weight, and can offer a guide as to optimum weight to aim for. Again, simple exercise, will reduce excess weight (coupled with a sensible diet) and will improve flexibility.

To reiterate, good physical fitness doesn't have to be a draconian regime of hard work and tiring exercise. Ideally, it is simple, natural exercise taken each day, and built to a daily routine. In a few days, the readers fitness will begin to drastically improve, and within weeks, he or she will forget they are even doing it! It's that simple!

A healthy fitness plan for healthy living doesn't have to be a tough grind every day. A short amount of exercise of medium intensity every day or at least every two days in three, is an excellent framework for building a good level of fitness. If possible, the plan should be combined with daily living and activities, of course for the first week or so, it will seem like an uphill battle, however, by the end of the first week, the activities will be noticeably easier, than when the activities were started. Inside of three weeks, the body will have adjusted to the 'new routine' of exercise and not only will it be relatively easy, but psychologically, it won't be perceived as a negative activity in the mind. In fact, after a short time, perhaps a month, the body will be so used to the endorphins being released in the brain due to exercise and getting outside in the sunshine and fresh air that the shooter will begin to miss 'not' doing their exercise.

So, there endeth the pep talk, now let's look at good exercise that reflects the typical daily physical activities of the traditional Japanese way of living that can be adapted to a Western lifestyle. Walking and swimming are all low impact exercises, which mimic our body's experience in the natural environment. These exercises are all high repetition, low power exercises that tend to improve cardio vascular and pulmonary fitness, as opposed to building muscle. Exercises such as weight lifting, squats, and treadmill/jogging exercise don't achieve the type of fitness (cardio vascular and pulmonary) required for all the disciplines of battlefield arts. Moreover, they are high impact exercises, and are not conducive to prolonging the life of joints in the body.

So where is a good place to start? Take simple walking for an example. We walk in everyday life, we walk at work and we walk when we are in our home environments, our body's are designed for walking and for most people, walking is a simple, low impact exercise. So, what better way to start on the path to a good fitness plan than walking down a path!

Initially, we need to do less than we think we should. If we go out and walk too much to begin with, we will end up with sore muscles, a lethargic state and sore feet. We should start off with small steps, perhaps take a walk, at a medium pace, around the equivalent of two city blocks, returning to the starting point or for 15 minutes. Take some music with along, as company. When we have finished, we will feel warm, slightly out of breath, but will recover well over a further 15 to 30 minutes. We need to do this for a week, and by the end of the week they will be covering the same distance, faster and with less effort. The start of week two is the time start stepping the intensity and distance. Try to walk around the equivalent of four city blocks or 30 minutes at a medium pace. Again, we will probably end up sweating slightly and be a little out of breath. The start of week three will have you in an established routine on an established route and getting used to the exercise. Any soreness you may have felt when starting the exercise plan will have faded and the walking that you do do will have become to feel fairly effortless. Now is the time to step up the pace to medium fast. Most people walk at roughly 4km per hour. This is slow. Try to aim for 6-7km per hour. If we can maintain this pace for a full 30 minutes, every day, we have set an excellent routine, that will see their cardio vascular and pulmonary fitness improve quickly and significantly, and will also develop a wide band of muscles that are directly useful in most daily activities.

It is important to address two key points when embarking on a fitness plan such as this however, firstly, for the first week, we is going to feel tired, sore and lethargic. This is because our body's are adapting its muscles, joints and biochemical processes to suit a new activity. It will hurt, and we won't want to do it, but we must push through it and keep going. Once we are into the second week, we will wonder what all the fuss is about. Secondly, now that we are changing the energy and hydration requirements of their body, we must address our diet and water intake to suit the activity. Finally, this system can be equally applied to swimming or cycling. Perhaps try cycling to work, or stopping at a public pool on the way home. Exercise itself is easy, possessing the psychology to carry through with exercise and be firm with oneself is hard and speaks to the sense of perseverance that we are trying to attain.

The outcome of following this diet will be that in amongst a frantically paced world, time is taken each day for the preservation and development of self, and over time strength of character, fitness, wisdom and well-being will result.

The Ninja

There are few warrior castes associated with individual cultures around the world better known that the *ninja*. However, the modern understanding of the ninja is the product of legend and popular culture, particularly in the West.

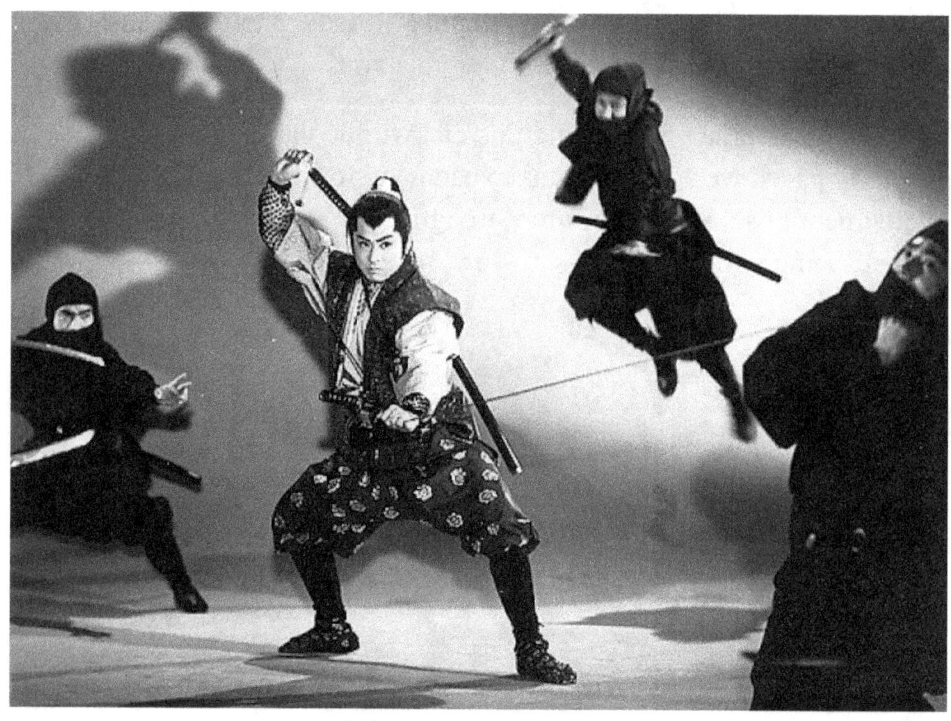

A contemporised and westernised view of the Ninja from the 1967 movie 'Red Shadow'.

There is little historical reference material available on the *ninja* and many historians have postulated various concepts and ideas on who the *ninja* were, how they lived and how they died. What is known is that there is a world of difference between the early accounts of mystics and druids who lived in the forests and mountains of the old Japan, as opposed to the more modern accounts that look upon the ninja as expertly trained, hired assassins. While the truth may never be known, there is a consensus of sorts, and that is where we will begin.

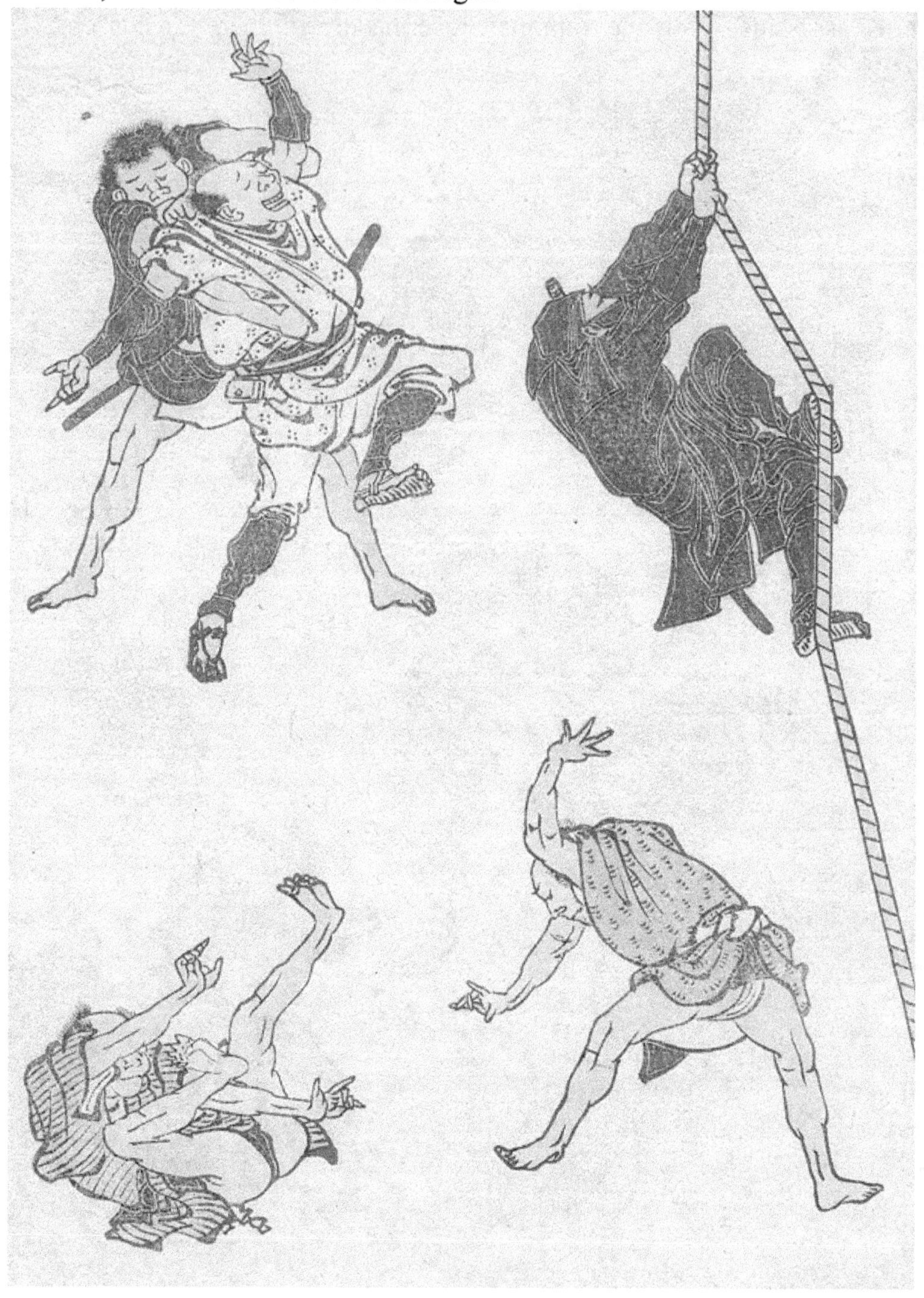

Early accounts speak of the agrarian lower classes in the feudal hierarchy where the local fisherman or farmer may, for a price, provide various acts associated with the *ninja* such as sabotage, reconnaissance and assassination. These people were a simple people leading a simple life, tied closely to the earth that sustained them, and utilised the tools they had available such as scythes, staves and nets. Later accounts speak more to the *ninja* as "Ronin" or displaced *Samurai* who would sell their services to the highest bidder, and possessed a higher level of martial training and ability.

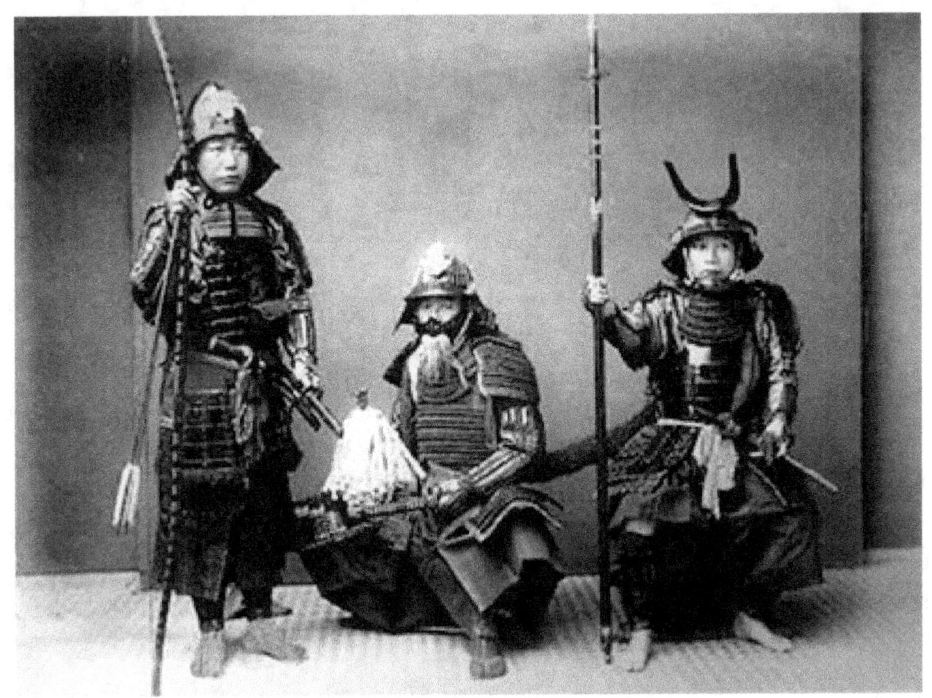

An early photo of a group of Samurai.

Both counts agree that the *ninja* were a people who persevered with limited resources, had little capacity to remain static and had to rely on their wits to survive. An unpredictable life lead in this way requires several key factors related to survival psychology, and these are; a capacity to self-regulate and remain calm, an ability to adapt and persevere when under stress, and wholesome diet to sustain the body that is constantly at a high state of readiness.

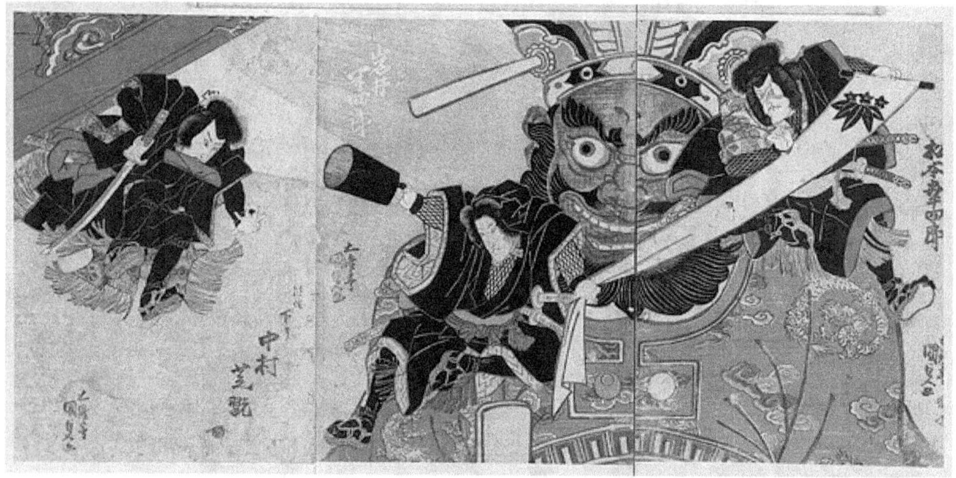

An 1820's woodblock depicting the perception of the Ninja in the Japanese psyche.

The modern world reflects many of these pressures upon all of us, and much like the ninja of old, we too can learn lessons to teach us how to persevere, adapt and overcome all the challenges that stare us down.

The Kuji-In

The *Kuji-In* or *Kuji-Kiri* is a meta-physical practice stemming from traditional Taoism in China, and again revolves traditionally around the number nine, although there is evidence to suggest that there are about 280 separate *Kuji-In*. The practice, in part requires that the practitioner perform various 'seals' or shapes with their hands to invoke the assistance of a Buddhist deity in pursuit of healing, power and other physical manifestations. This practice was heavily used and continues to be used by Shugendo priests and '*Yamabushi*' or mountain hermits. It was not unknown for these *Yamabushi* to fight alongside *Samurai* during times of unrest and this may be how these practices found their association with *Ninja*.

ZEN	ZAI	RETSU	JIN	KAI	SHA	TOH	PYO	RIN
前	在	裂	陳	皆	者	闘	兵	臨
隠形印	日輪印	智拳印	内縛印	外縛印	内師子印	外師子印	大金剛輪印	獨古印

The commonly recognised Kuji-in hand seals - although history tells us there are far more than nine.

Popular culture sees the *Kuji-In* as a more mystical or dark art and akin to Western idea's of witchcraft and spell casting. Myths tell us of the use of *Kuji-In* for the performing of incredible acts such as turning invisible or bringing the dead back to life, and it is common for a people in the absence of science to explain the inexplicable, as magic.

The truth of the *Kuji-In* lies somewhere closer to the centre, and in determining where the truth lies we need to consider that translations of Asian languages are highly interpretive. It may be true that a warrior hiding from an enemy performed one of the *Kuji-In* and was not detected, and a legend was born – but this is far from turning invisible and speaks more to the concept of faith and the Taoist roots of the *Kuji-In*.

If one sets aside the more spiritual aspects of the *Kuji-In* and looks to psychological science for answers, we can determine some psychological and physiological changes occur when the *Kuji-In* are performed. The amygdala is an evolutionally older portion of each brain hemisphere that is closely linked to emotional learning, the fight or flight response and memory creation. The amygdalae, together with the rest of the limbic portions of the brain define and control emotional responses to stimuli, and act autonomically as a defence mechanism. Unfortunately, this response can be counterproductive as it does not involve any moderation from the neocortex or the cognitive and thinking centres of the brain. The amygdalae being a learning structure can be both calmed and conditioned and it is well known that the sense of 'inner calm' experienced by yoga practitioners, those who meditate and those who 'loose themselves' in a task or activity experience a calming of the amygdalae. Performing of the *Kuji-In*, sometimes with concentration and chanting achieves the same physiological response within the brain and the psychological calming that result from it. This act can be highly centering and grounding for a person who is beginning to mentally dysregulate, and when repeated teaches the brain to regulate the amygdalae responses to stimuli which would otherwise cause a sense of fear, anxiety or distress.

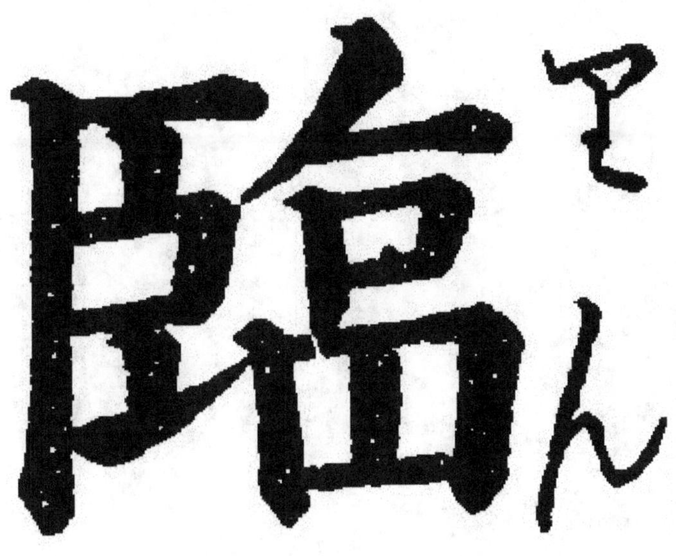

Rin – Power – Directedness of Thought

To perform this *Kuji-in* the practitioner interlocks their fingers of each hand much like a double fist, leaving their middle fingers extended forming a triangle.

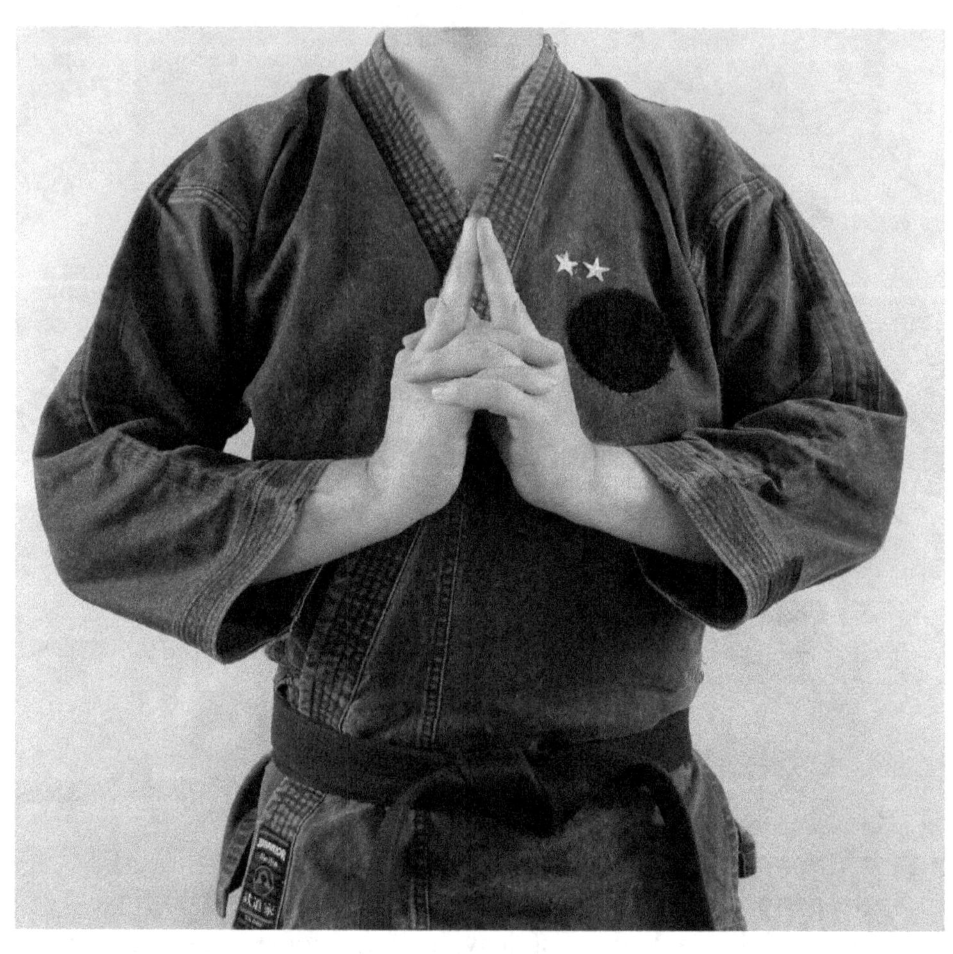

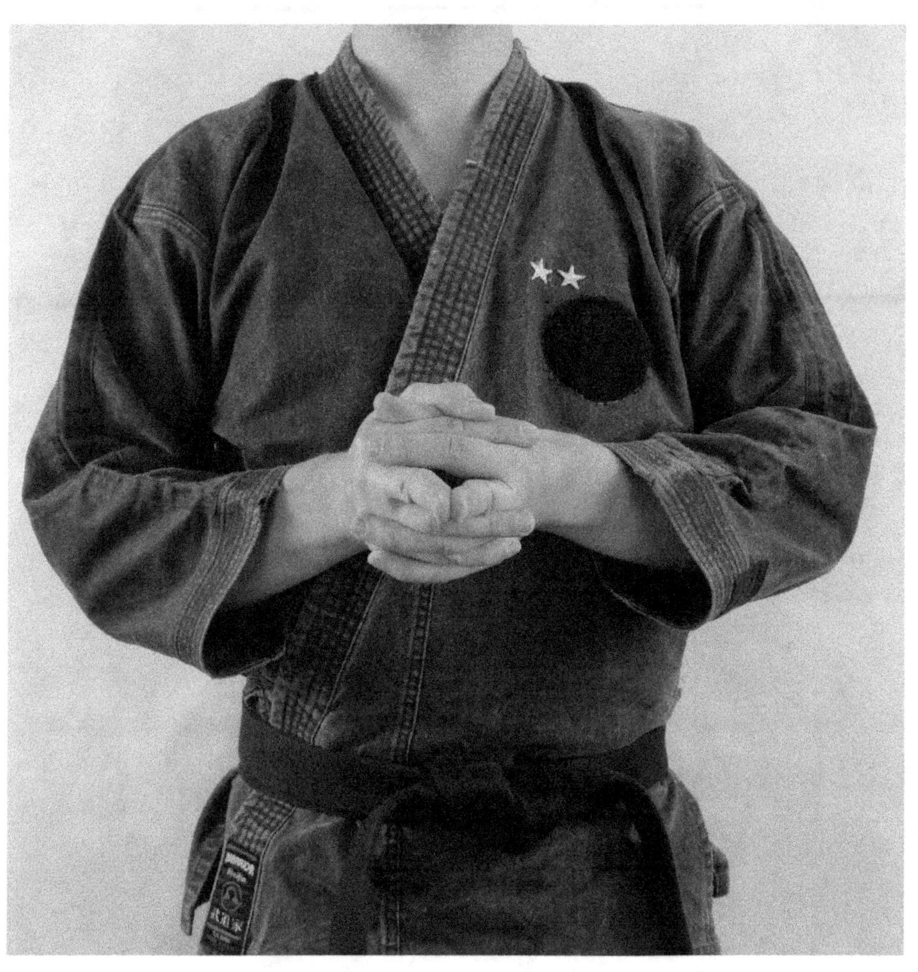

Haiku

No one travels
Along this way but I,
This autumn evening.

\- Matsuo Bashō

Legend

Kido Yazaemon was born in Tenbun 8, 1539 in the mountains of Iga prefecture. His early years focussed on the *Ikko* religion. The *Ikko-Ikki* religion was a sect of peasants and farmers who engaged in Buddhist worship of *Amida*. This sect was isolationist and pursued a more aggressive reading of the teachings of *Shinran* and were known to engage in collective practices for self determination and defence. While these small isolated sects posed no military threat to the *Shogunate* and local *Daimyo*, their existence posed a socio-political threat to rule in the feudal system. Kido Yazaemon grew up living in an armed camp and it was through this experience and training that he learned his martial skills, as well as resilience, resourcefulness and field craft, which would all serve him to great effect in later life.

The *Ikko-Ikki* pursued limited armed conflict and were a irregular force used by both Oda Nobunaga and Tokugawa Ieyasu at various times and won some victories most notably at the Battle of Kuzuryugawa and the Battle of Sendanno. Typically the *Ikko-Ikki* would go into battle with limited armour, wearing monks robes and carrying various banners reflecting their faith. Armaments consisted primarily of the *Naginata*, a four to six *shaku* (foot) pole with a one *shaku* curved blade at the end, although other weapons, including rudimentary firearms in the form of Portuguese Arbequesses were available.

Kido Yazaemon favoured the Arbequess and was known to be an excellent shot. In the year of 1579, Kido Yazaemon attempted an assassination of Oda Nobunaga, due to Nobunaga's pursuit of the *Ikko-Ikki* and subsequent invasion and destruction of Nagashima Castle. Kido Yazaemon remained behind as *Ikko-Ikki* forces retreated and early one morning while Oda Nobunaga was inspecting his forces following a skirmish, Kido Yazaemon sprung his trap. Although Kido Yazaemon failed to kill Oda Nobunaga he did succeed in killing seven of Oda Nobunaga's bodyguards and successfully turned the axis of advance of Oda Nobunaga's forces to allow for the *Ikko-Ikki* to withdraw.

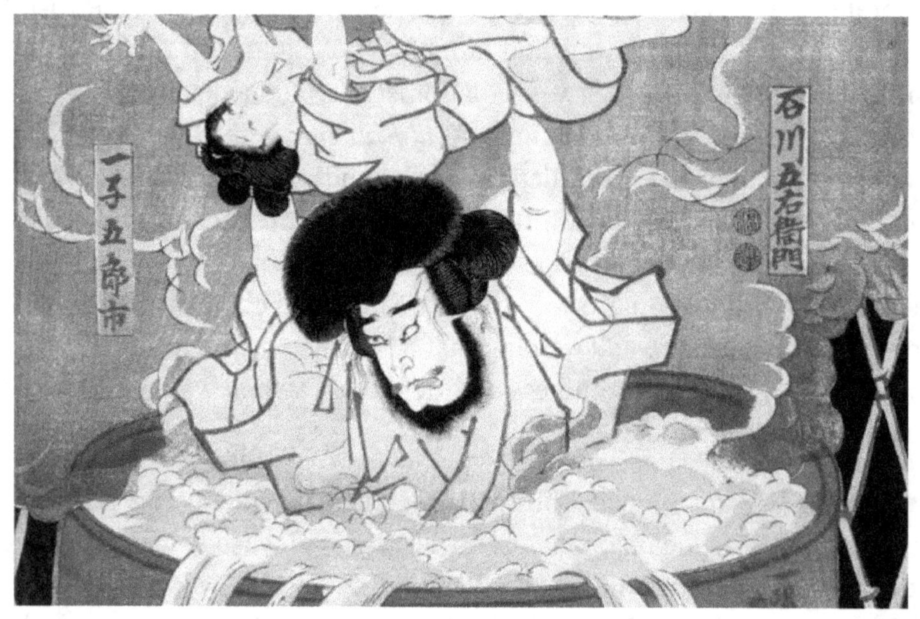

Popular image of Kido Yazaemon as he and his son were executed.

Recipe: Hyorougan

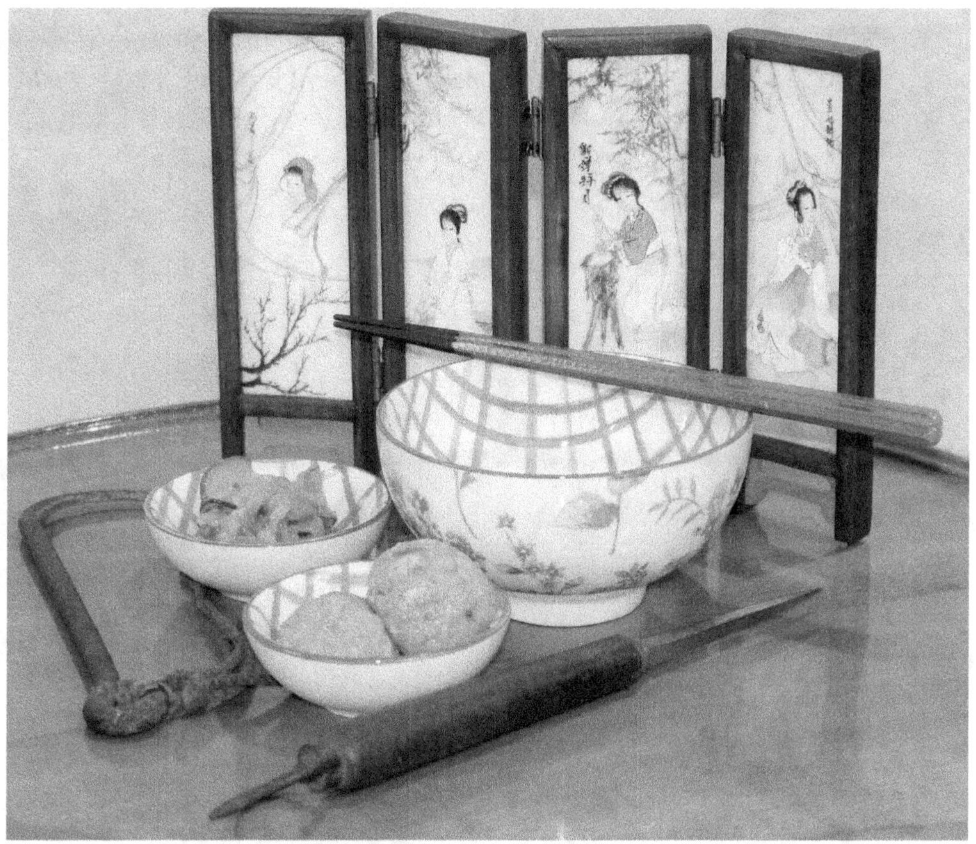

Hyorougans were considered to be the MRE (Meal- Ready to Eat) of the *Ninja*. The recipe varied on the availability of some ingredients however it was considered to be a sustaining, medicinal and used for bursts of physical and mental strength and energy.

- Glutinous Rice – 60 parts
- Rice – 60 parts
- Lotus Seed – 1 part

- Yam – 1 part
- Cinnamon – 1 part
- Coix Seed – 1 part
- Ginseng – 1 part
- Brown Sugar – 60 parts

Mix the ingredients with water to make a firm dough. Roll in to 1" balls. Steam in a basket steamer for approximately five minutes and allow to cool and dry off.

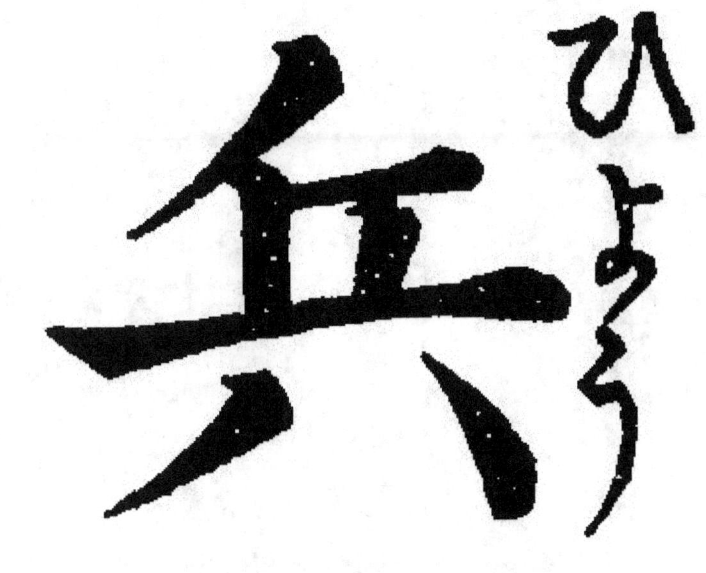

Pyo – Energy – Focus of Physical Strength

To perform this *Kuji-in* the practitioner interlocks the little and ring fingers of each hand, bring the index finger together in the form of a triangle and threat the middle fingers over the triangle bringing them back to touch the tips of the thumbs.

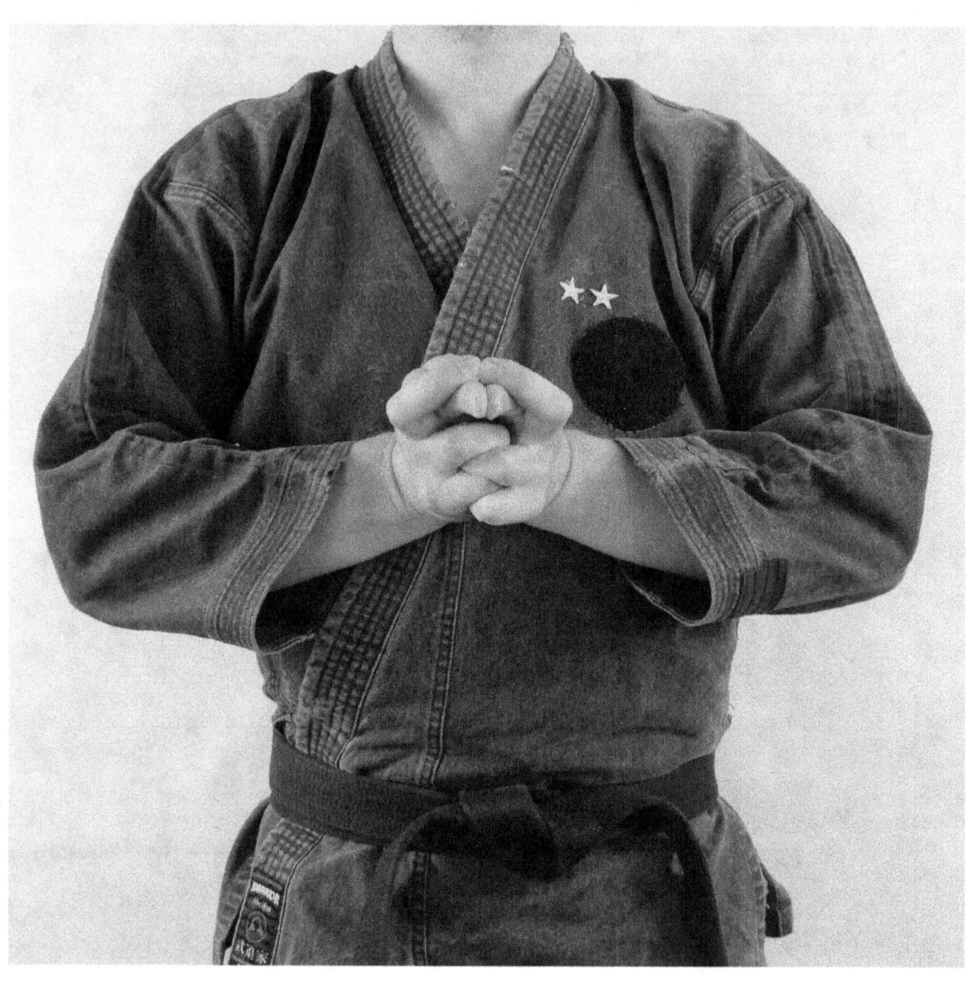

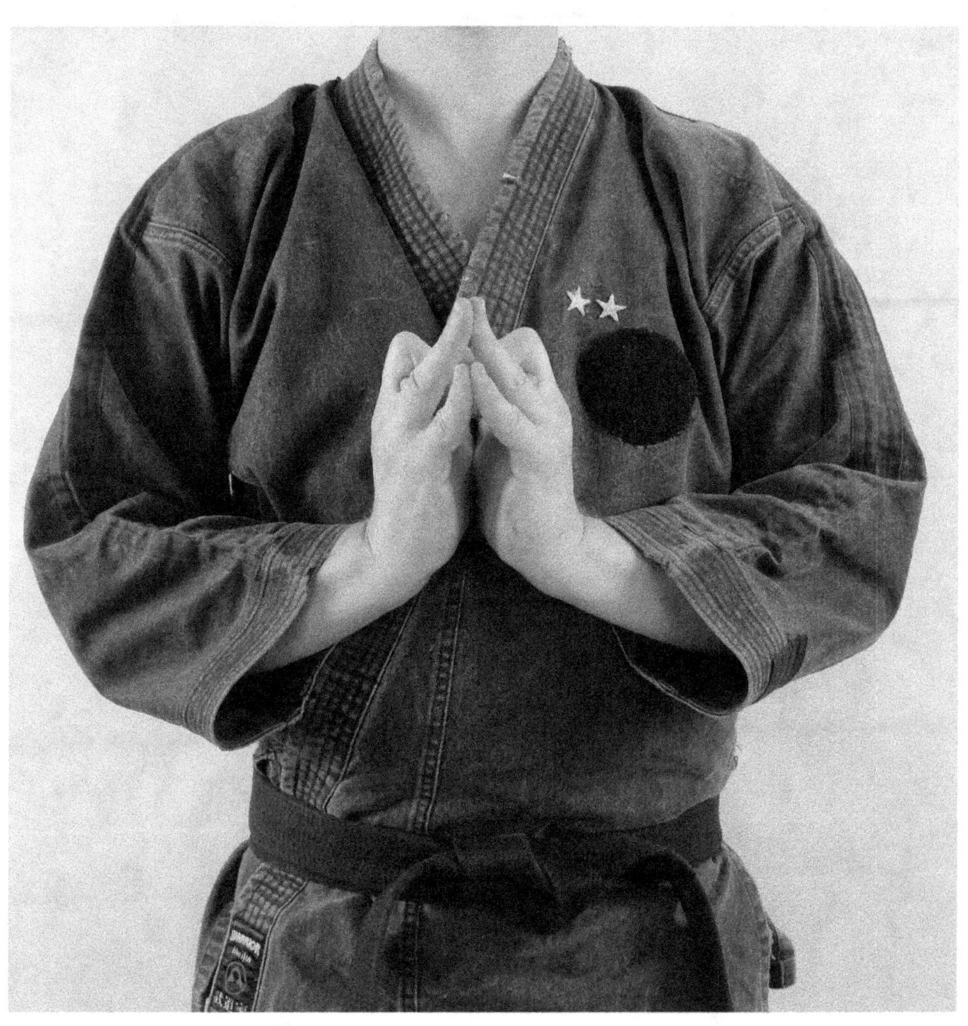

Haiku

*First autumn morning
the mirror I stare into
shows my father's face.*

- Murakami Kijo

Legend

During the Sengoku period Oda Nobunaga fought against Imagawa Yoshimoto for control of Owari prefecture and the status of most powerful Daimyo or warlord. Although Imagawa Yoshimoto was ultimately defeated and he himself killed at the battle of Okehazama for several years following Oda Nobunaga continued to engage remnant forces allied to Imagawa Yoshimoto.

During 1562 relatives of Nobunaga and Ieyasu were taken hostage by Imagawa Yoshimoto supporters and imprisoned at Kaminogu Castle under command of Udono Nagamochi – a general of some renown and closely tied to the Imagawa clan. Nobunaga and Ieyasu understanding the danger that their relatives were in looked towards Iga prefecture for assistance from the *Yamabushi*.

Tomo Sukesada, *Soke* or head of Tomo Ryu in Koga prefecture was engaged by Oda Nobunaga and Tokugawa Ieyasu to infiltrate the castle and rescue the family members who now even included Tokugawa Ieyasu's wife and child son. Tomo Sukesada assembled a force of 80 Koga *Ninja* and observed the castle for many days, learning the routines of the guards, passwords and clothing used.

In the late evening the *Ninja* force infiltrated the castle by using stealth and deception and quickly took control of the outer defences setting fire to the towers as a diversion to allow a smaller group, including Tokugawa Ieyasu himself, and another Ninja of renown, Hattori Hanzo with Tomo Sukesada to go in search of the hostages. During the search this smaller force was intercepted by Udono Nagamochi and his bodyguards. A desperate struggle ensued and ultimately Udono Nagamochi was killed and the hostages rescued before the Imagawa forces could rally.

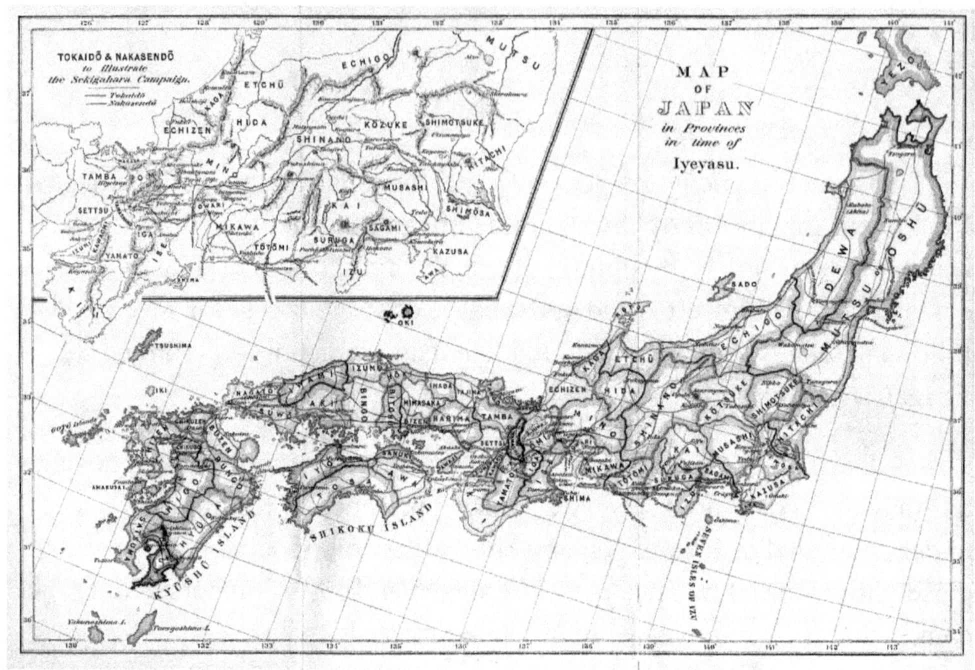

The historical provinces of Japan.

Recipe: Kikatsugan

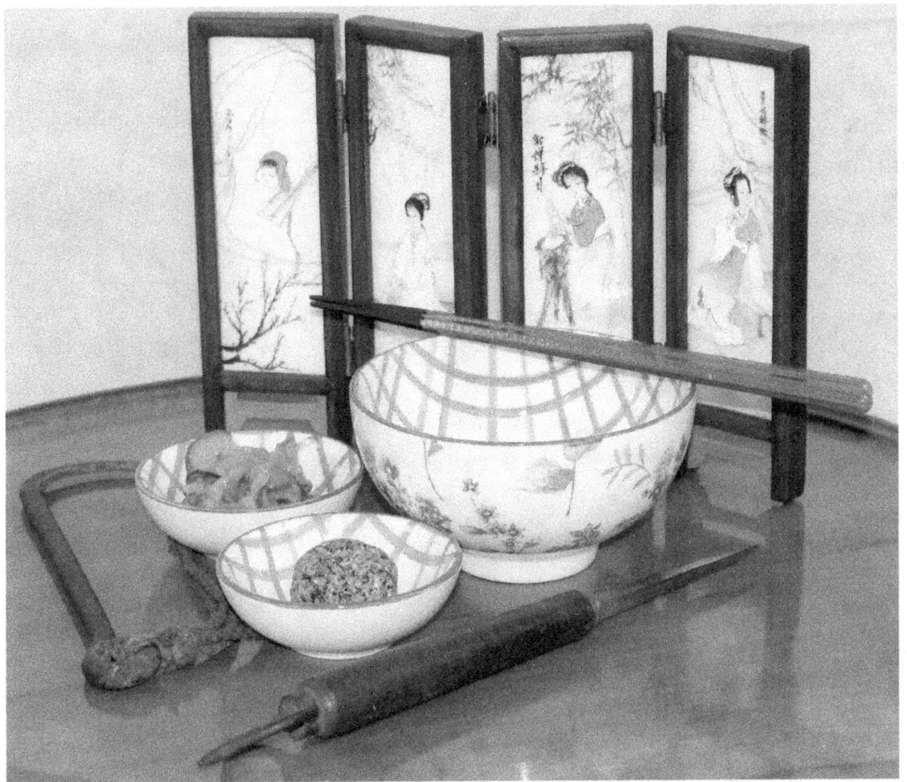

Kikatsugan is another military field ration that can be eaten in place of a main meal. The original recipe required that the ingredients be soaked in *Sake* or Japanese rice wine for three years however this is open to interpretation.

- Carrots – 10 parts

- Buckwheat – 20 parts

- Wheat – 20 parts

- Yams – 20 parts

- Licorice – 1 part

- Barley – 10 parts

- Glutinous Rice – 20 parts

The ingredients are simply kneaded together with water and rolled into small plum sized balls and allowed to air dry.

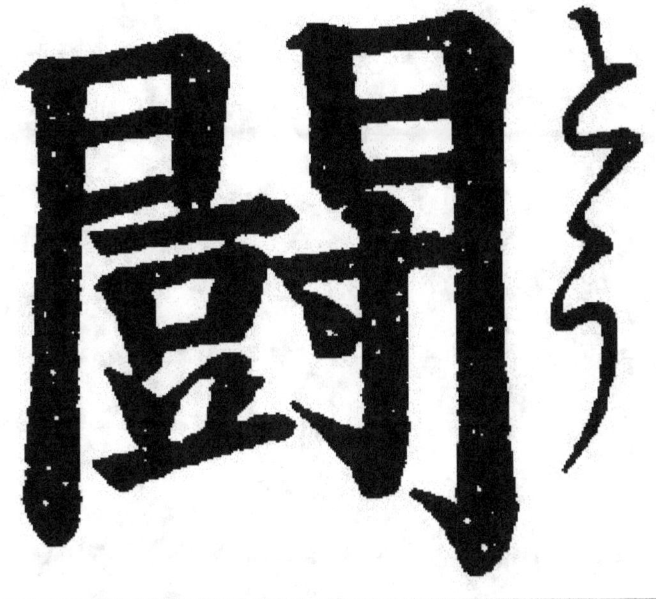

To – Harmony – Internal Balance and Calm

To perform this *Kuji-in* the practitioner extends the little and ring fingers of each hand and allows them to touch at the tips forming two triangles. The index fingers are crossed over each other and allow the middle fingers to wrap down over them. The thumbs are simply placed alongside each other.

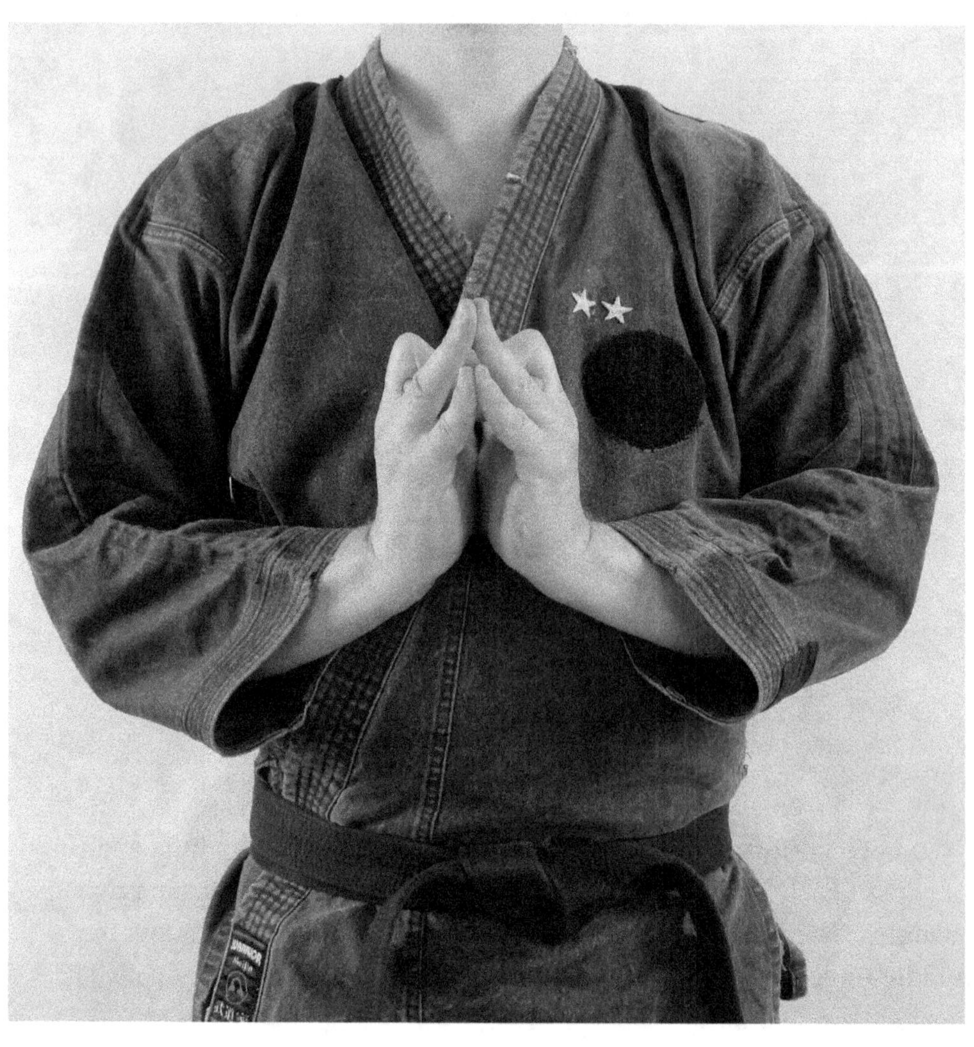

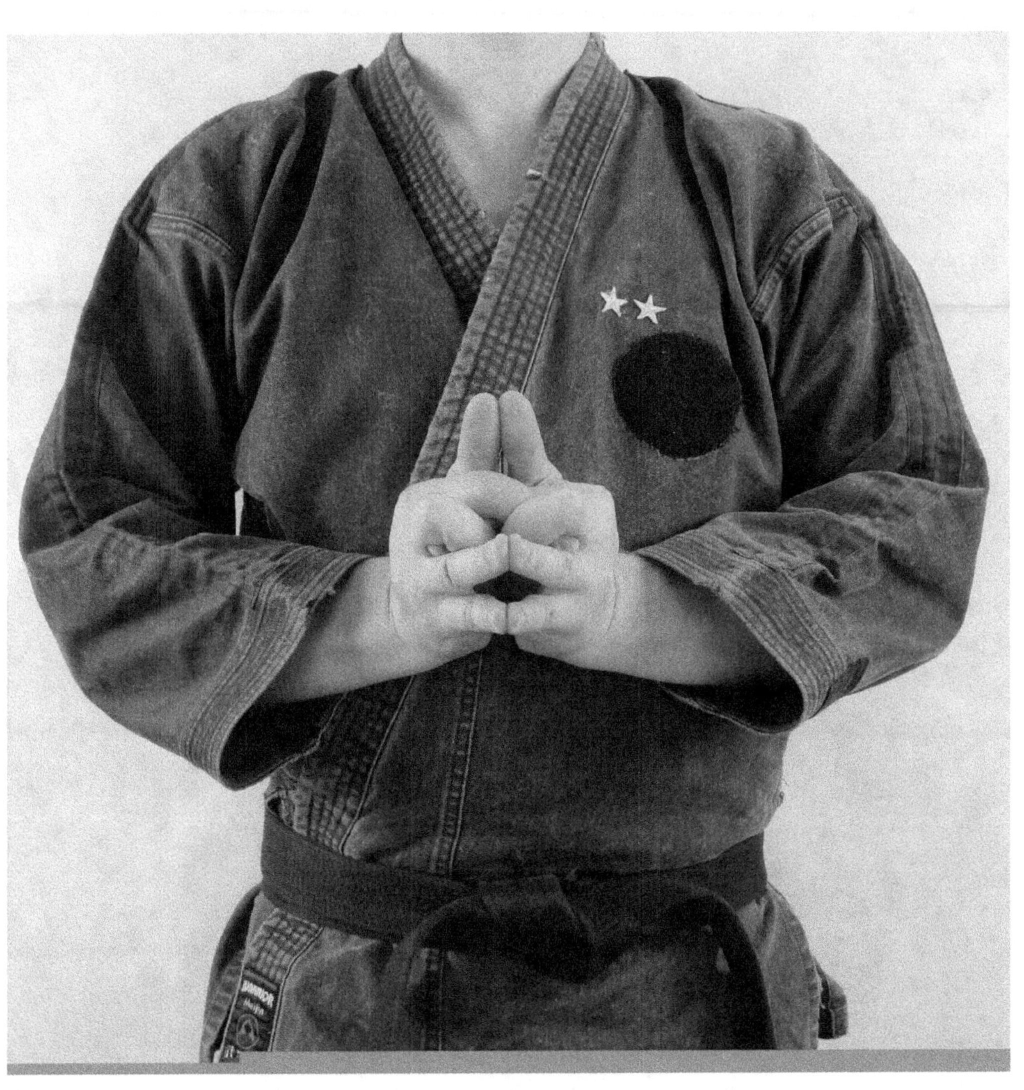

Haiku

*Winter seclusion -
Listening, that evening,
To the rain in the mountain.*

\- Kobayashi Issa

Legend

Fujibayashi Nagato was something of an enigma, part legend and part myth the truth around Fujibayashi Nagato may never be fully known. What is known however is that Fujibayashi was one of the great *Ninja* of the Sengoku period from 1467-1603 and otherwise known as the Warring States period. Fujibayashi Nagato lived in the northern part of the Iga province and is known to have collaborated with both Hattori Hanzo and Momochi Sandayu to train, equip and engage Iga *Ninja* in *Shinobi* activities. Some sources suggest that Fujibayashi Nagato and Momochi Sandayu were in fact the same person, and the change in names was a deception designed to strengthen the sense of durability for those who might consider to attempt to annihilate the Iga clans.

In early 1581, two Iga *Ninja* realised the notoriety that Iga *Ninja* beginning to receive and the resultant risks that were building and travelled to Azuchi and defected to Oda Nobunaga, providing critical information and offering to act as guides in return for the safety of their families. With this agreement in place and with the assistance of the defectors, in mid 1581 Oda Nobunaga invaded the Iga prefecture with upwards of 42,000 men under eight generals and commenced the second Tensho Iga war.

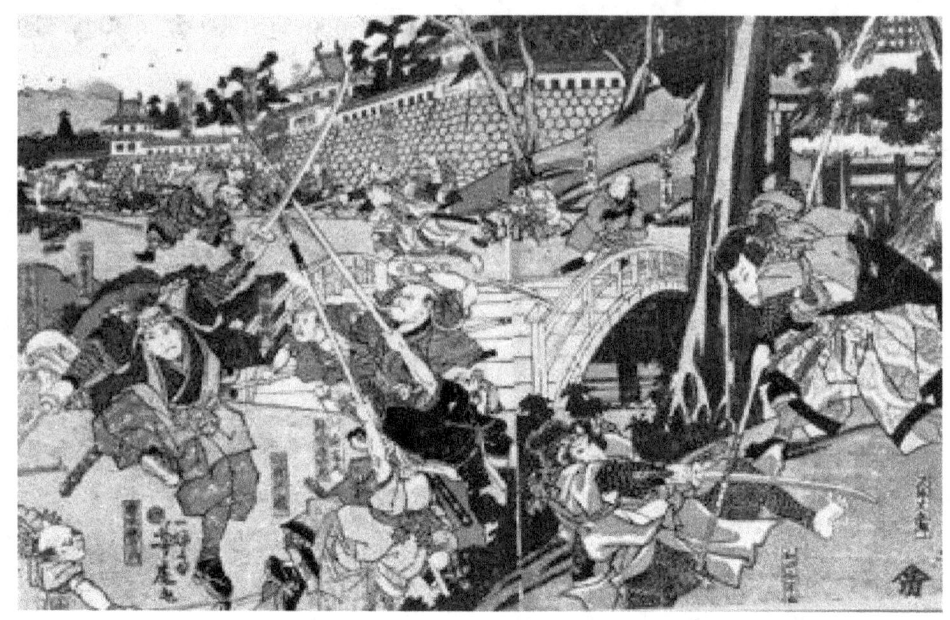

Early woodblock depicting the Tensho Iga war of 1581.

Given the geographical separation of the Iga prefecture and the mountainous terrain, Fujibayashi Nagato was only able to gather a force of approximately 10,000 men, and although Fujibayashi Nagato was ultimately defeated and killed along with the bulk of Iga forces, he did take a small group, infiltrate Oda Nobunaga's lines and kill the two defectors, and their families before withdrawing to the shadows of history.

Today, we know of Fujibayashi Nagato primarily from the writings of the *Bansenshukai* or book of training for *Shinobi* and *Ninja*, that was compiled in the late 1600's by the remnants of the Fujibayashi clan.

Recipe: Suikatsugan

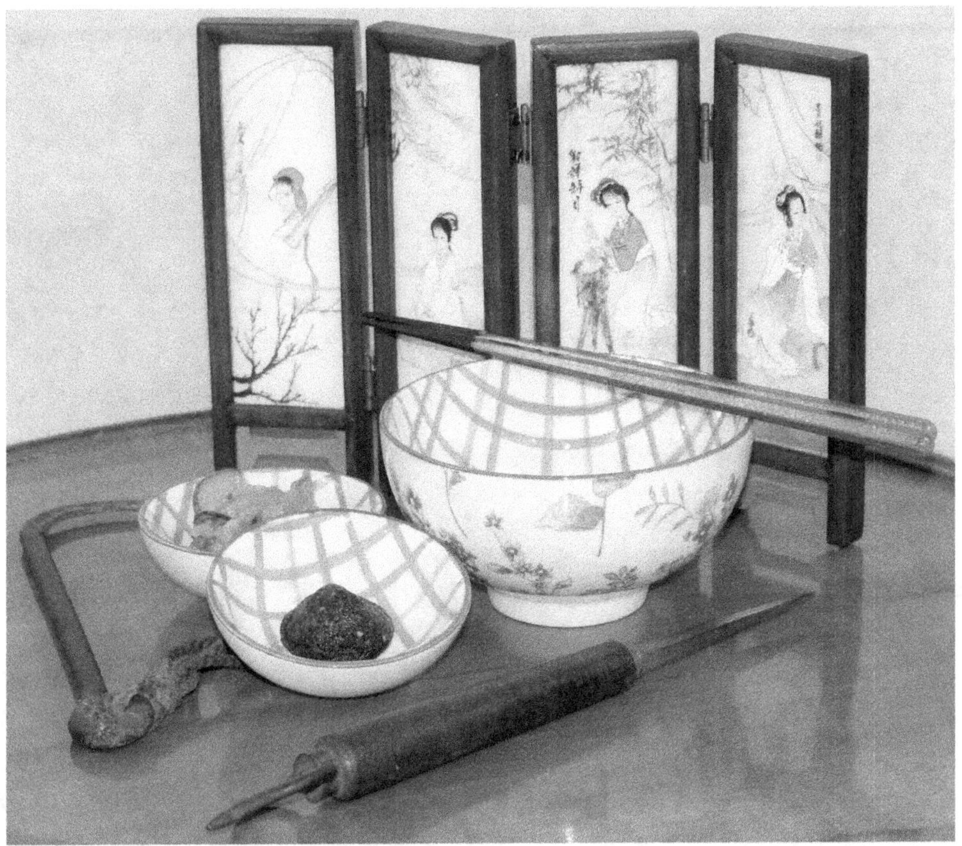

Suikatsugan is traditionally thought of as a thirst quenching and hunger relieving herbal medicine but was also used as chewing gum might be used in contemporary society.

- Pickled Plum – 8 parts

- Rock Sugar – 2 parts

- Powdered Ergot – 1 part

The ingredients are simply kneaded together with water into cherry sized balls and allowed to air dry.

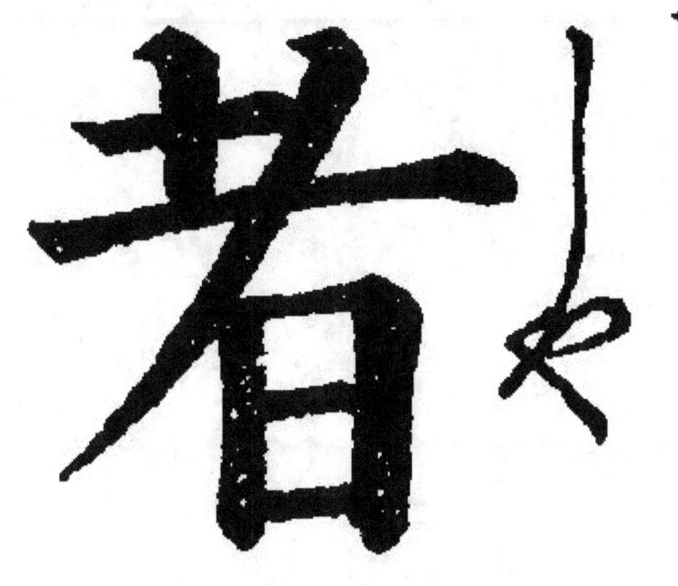

Sha – Healing – Mindfulness of Body

To perform this *Kuji-in* the practitioner extends the little fingers of each hand and allows them to touch at the tips forming two triangles. The ring fingers are crossed over each other and allow the middle fingers to wrap down over them. The index fingers are extended and allowed to touch at the tips forming a triangle. The thumbs are simply placed alongside each other.

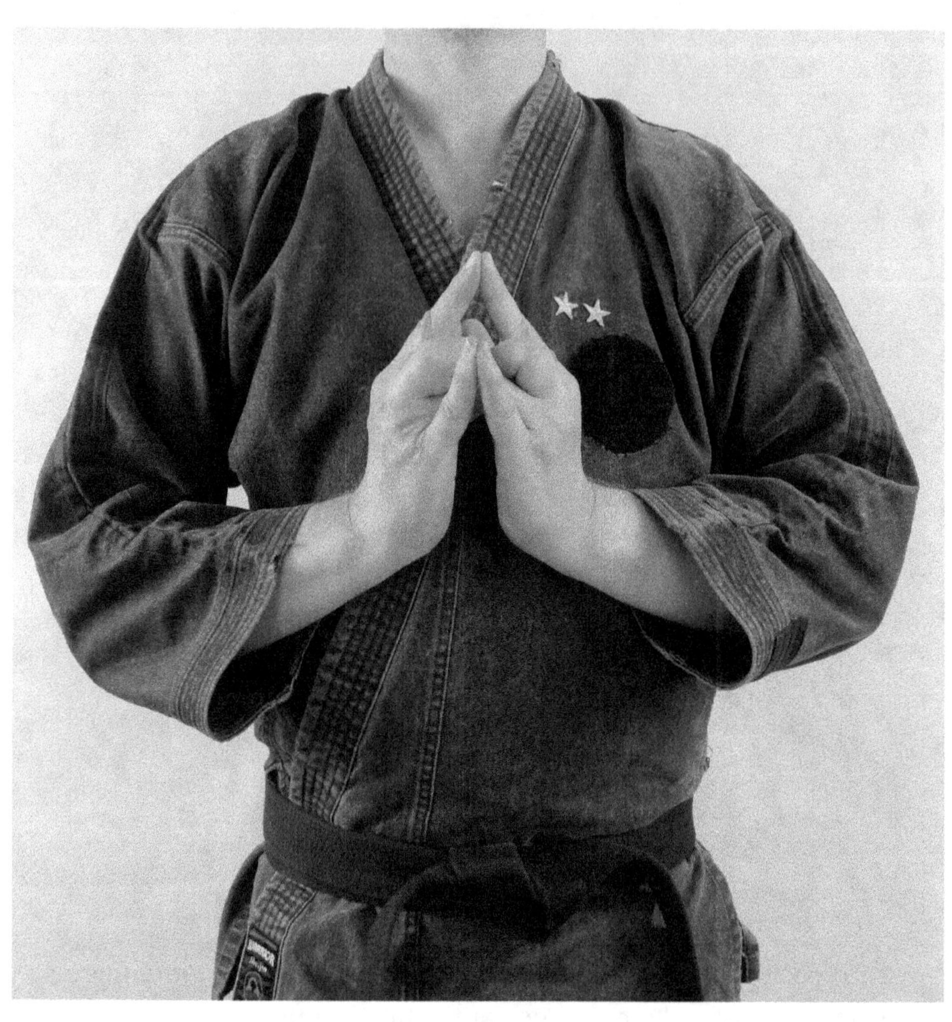

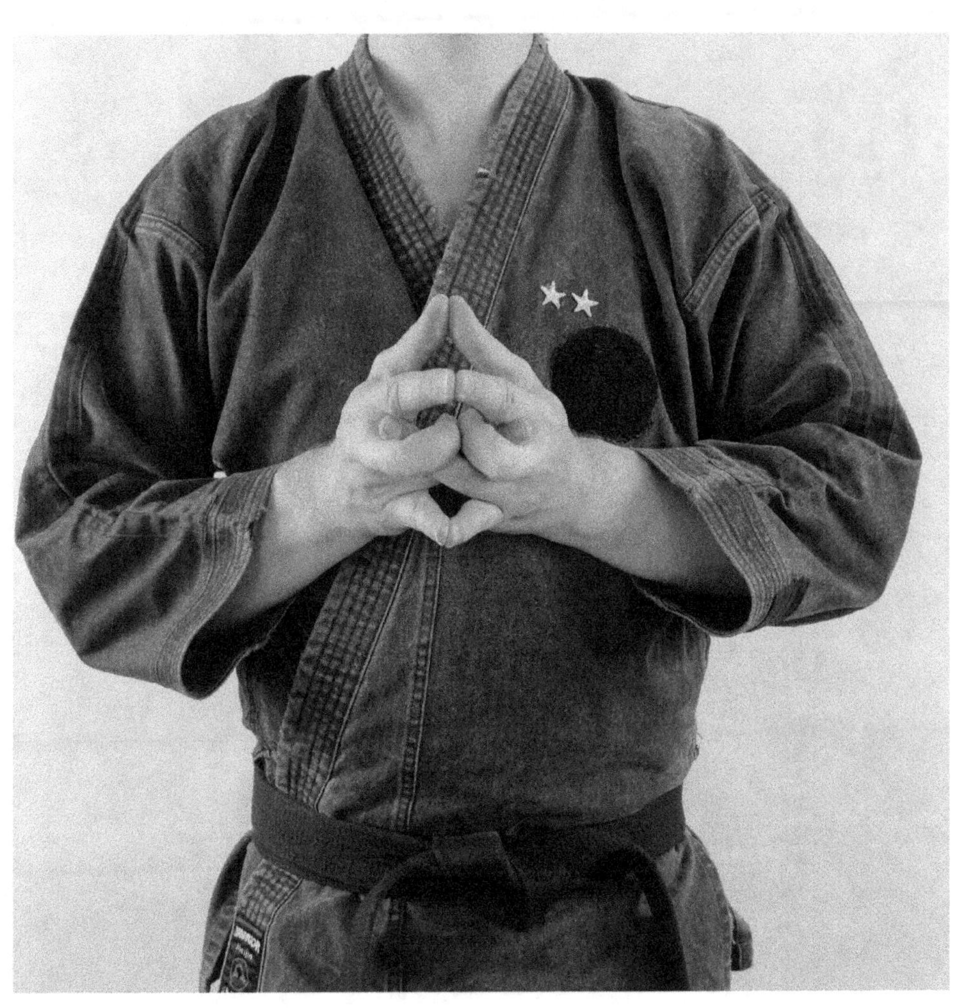

Haiku

*The wren
Earns his living
Noiselessly.*

- Kobayahsi Issa

Legend

In the annals of history there also existed female *Ninja*, or *Kunoichi* who combined lethality with beauty. Mochizuki Chiyome was one of these *Kunoichi* who was active during the Sengoku period. There is a level on controversy around Mochizuki Chiyome – some scholars believe she existed, others believe the history has been corrupted, others yet still believe she did exist however she was Mochizuki Nobumasa, her purported husband, in disguise. Although the truth will never now be known there is a legend that can guide us.

Mochizuki Chiyome was a noblewoman married to Mochizuki Nobamasa, and a decendent of Mochizuki Izumonokama – a noted Koga *Ninja* of the 1400's. Around 1561, Mochizuki Nobamasa was killed in battle, and Mochizuki Chiyome passed into the care of Mochizuki Nobamasa's uncle – Takeda Shingen, a Daimyo of note who was battling the forces of Oda Nobunaga. Takeda Shingen, know of Mochizuki Chiyome's ancestral Iga past, tasked her with creating an all female *Ninja* or *Kunoichi* force who Takeda Shingen could use as special spies and assassins.

Mochizuki Chiyome set up her base of operations in the village of Nazu in the Shinshu area and recruited orphans, prostitutes and widows to learn the skills of spies and assassins and then take on disguises of *Geisha* or courtesans and priestesses to conduct their missions. It is expectedly unclear what tasks specifically were undertaken however at one point the network that was created spanned a wide area and over 300 agents. Likely work would have been as spies, seductresses and assassins.

The end of Mochizuki Chiyome is equally unclear however we to know that her benefactor Takeda Shingen died under mysterious circumstances in 1573 – it is possible that Mochizuki Chiyome found a

greater benefactor in Takeda Shingen's sympathetic enemies – Oda
Nobunaga and Tokugawa Ieyasu who were known to utilise Koga *Ninja*.

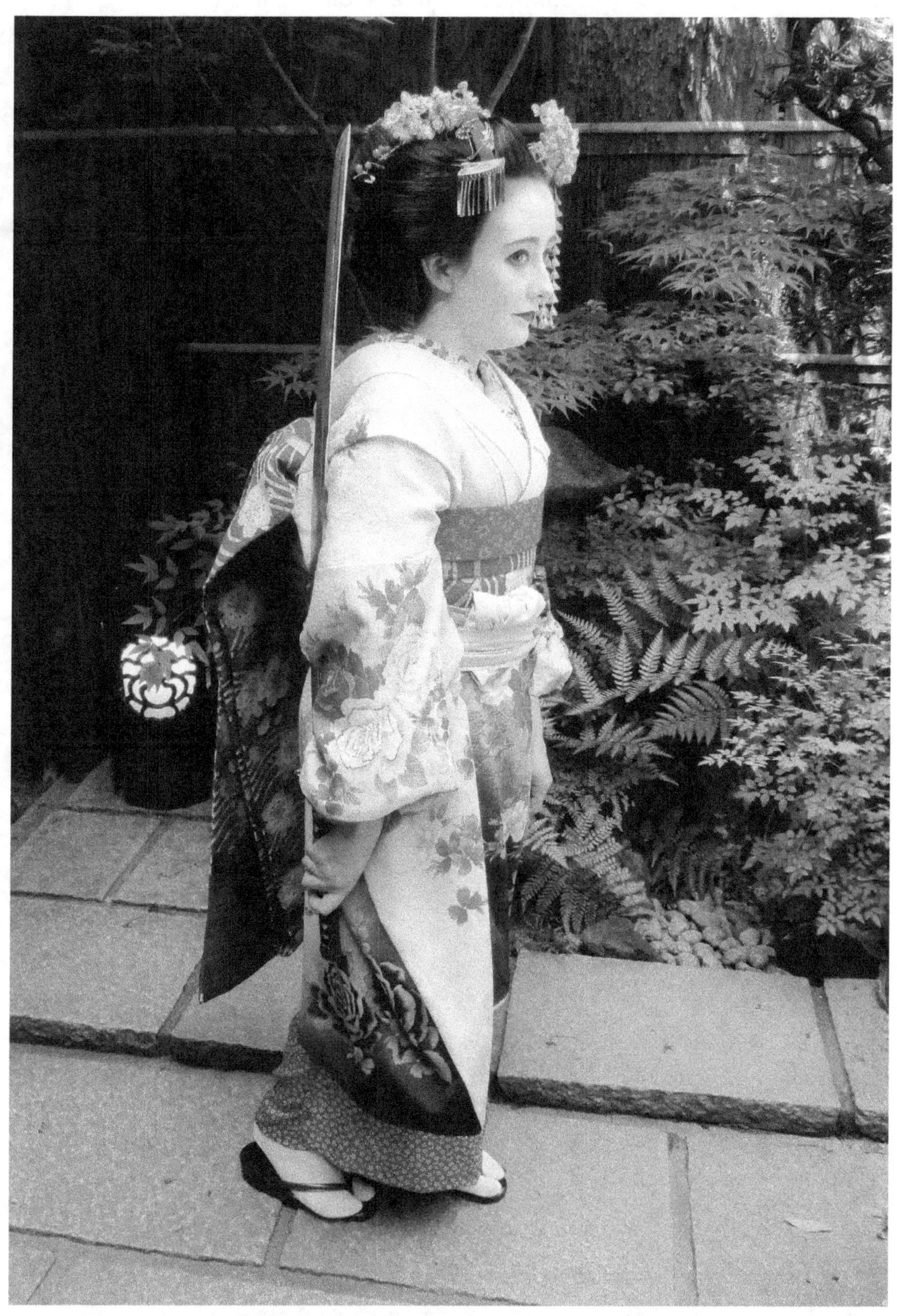

Death can walk in many forms.

Recipe: Chirinabe

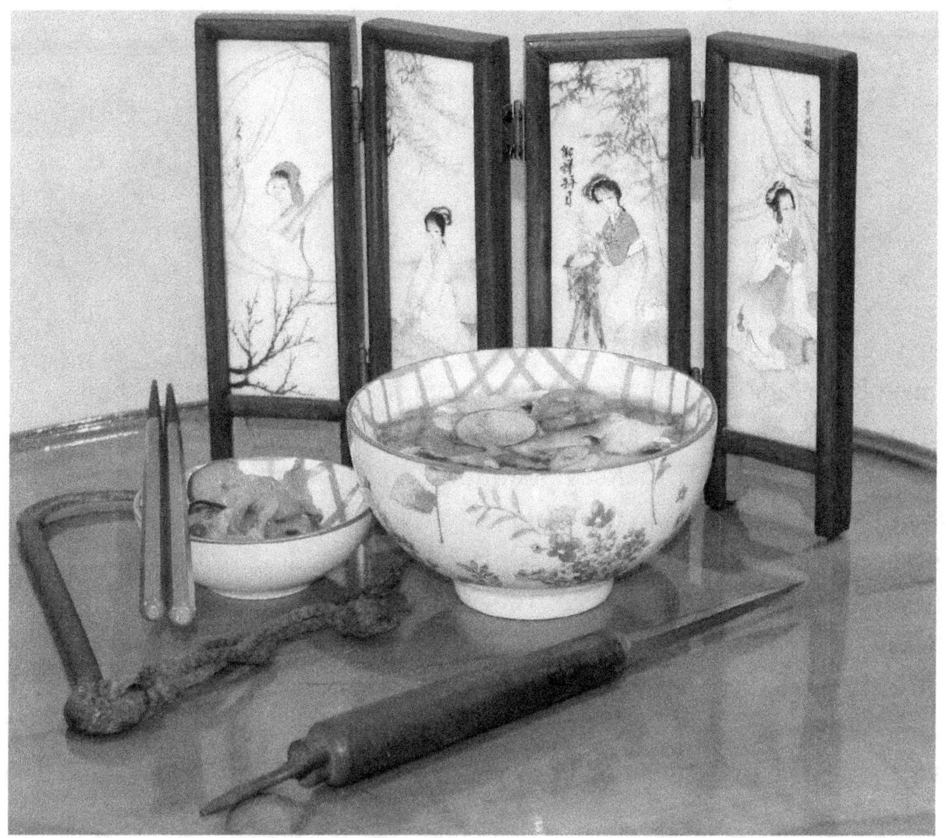

Chirinabe has its roots in the seaside communities of Mie Prefecture where the mountainous terrain limited agriculture and promoted a coastal fishing industry. Although Chirinabe today really only uses fish, any type of seafood can be used including hard shell crustaceans. The difference between Chirinabe and other hot pots is that Chirinabe focuses on communal eating and cooking.

- Seafood – 1 part

- Mushroom – 1 part

- Daikom Radish – 1 part

- Spring Onion – 1 part

- Dashi – 1 part

- Water – 4 parts

- Katsuobushi or Bonita Flakes – ½ part

- Mirin – ½ part

- Soy Sauce – ¼ part

The water is brought to the boil and Dashi, Mirin, Soy and Katsuobushi added. This is then simmered for five minutes and then strained. The vegetables are thinly sliced and added to the boiling broth and simmered for a further seven minutes. Following this the seafood in small pieces is brought to the table raw and the boiling broth on a small burner to maintain a rolling boil is placed in the middle of the table. Each guest then selects various pieces of seafood and adds them to the broth cooking them individually to taste and then combines with the vegetables and broth in a small bowl. Although seafood is traditionally used, a common variation is to use ground chicken, pork or beef in meatballs, and the cook in the same way. Also soba or udon noodles can also be added to the broth.

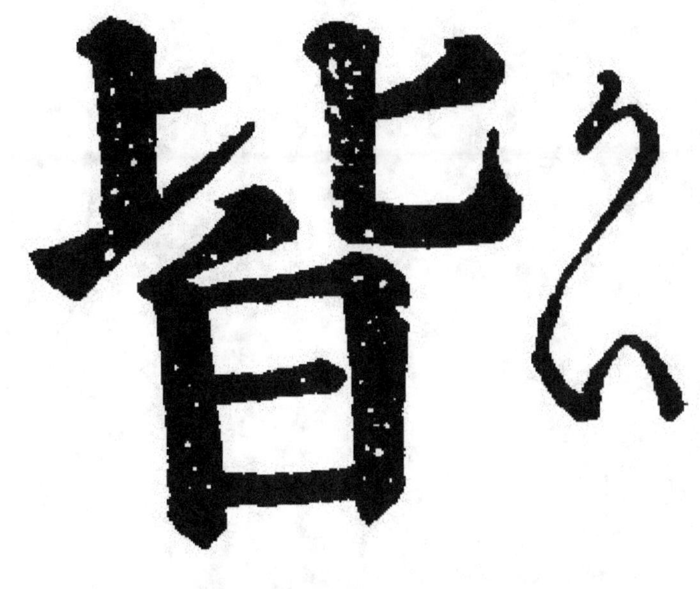

Kai – Intuition – Situational Intelligence

To perform this *Kuji-in* the practitioner interlocks and crosses over all the fingers and thumbs with the fingers and thumbs remaining on the outside of the hands.

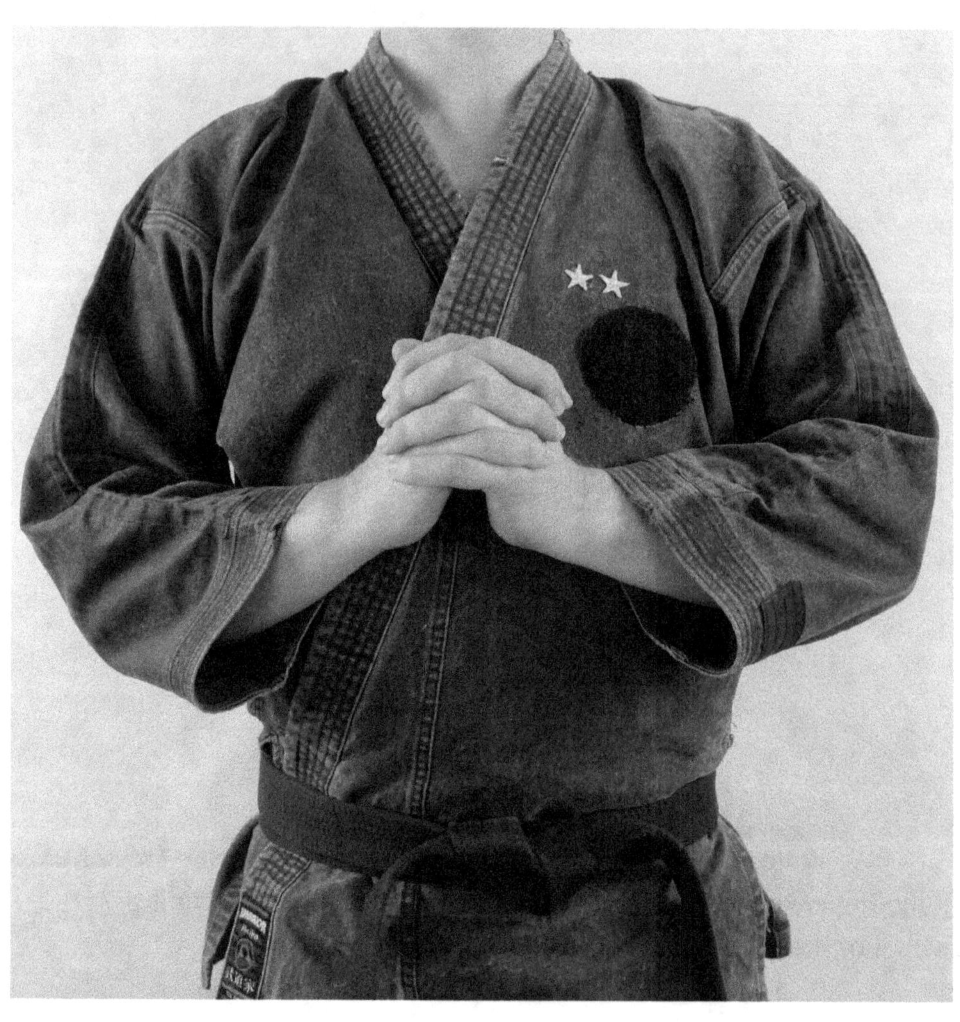

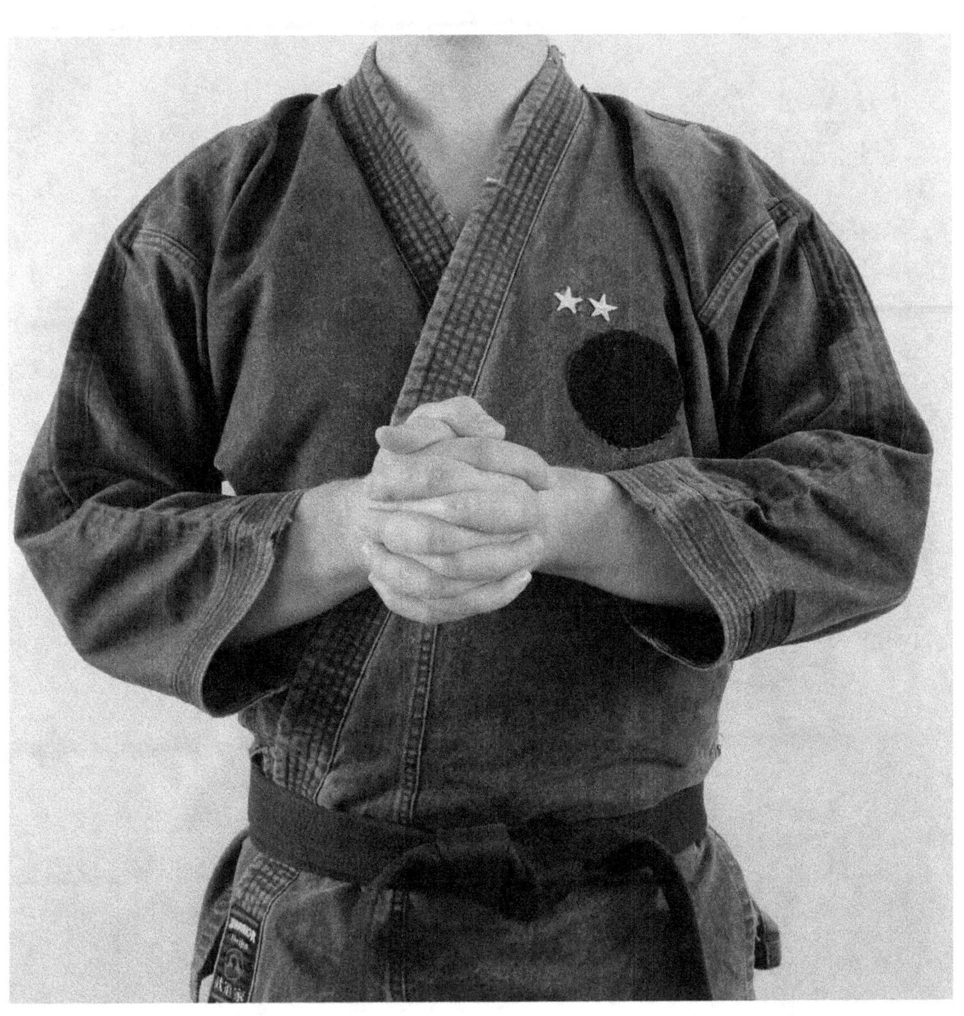

Haiku

*Over the wintry
forest, winds howl in rage
with no leaves to blow.*

- Natsume Soseki

Legend

Ishikawa Goemon is a figure as much of history as modern popular culture. Depending on the source Ishikawa Goemon is either portrayed as an honourable bandit or brave *Ninja* assassin. Ishikawa Goemon was born in 1558 to an honourable *Samurai* family in Iga prefecture and until age 15 lived a peaceful life. In 1573, Samurai of the Ashikaga *Shogunate* attacked and murdered his father for an unspecified transgression and Ishikawa Goemon was forced to flee with the remanants of his family.

Ishikawa Goemon came upon Momochi Sandayu and commenced training as an Iga *Ninja* in order to avenge his family. When the time was right, Ishikawa Goemon left his teacher and travelled into the world settling in the Kansai area where he used his *Shinobi* skills to support himself and soon found himself as the head man of a group of bandits against Toyotomi Hideyoshi where delving into his *Samurai* roots he would steal from the rich and give to the poor.

This continued for some years as Ishikawa Goemon contemplated his revenge. Toyotomi Hideoshi became aware of Ishikawa Goemon's activities and during a raid managed to kill Ishikawa Goemon's wife and capture his infant son and this was the catalyst that brought Ishikawa Goemon down.

In 1594 Ishikawa Goemon developed a plan to enter Fushimi castle and assassinate Toyotomi Hideyoshi, and late in that year he did so by himself. Managing to gain entry to the castle by night and sneaking across nightingale floors he managed to enter Toyotomi Hideyoshi's personal quarters, and only yards from his target he disturbed a bell that alerted the guards and after a brief struggle was captured.

Ishikawa Goemon was tried as a criminal and a bandit, in spite of his *Samurai* roots and was publicly boiled alive with his infant son.

Legend says that he held his son above his head until he began to succumb to his injuries and then plunged his son deep into the waters to quicken his death.

Ishikawa is portrayed as something of a folk hero in Japanese culture and there are many versions of his life and death, while there are conflicting views, what is clear is the Ishikawa Goemon is a victim of circumstance and honour.

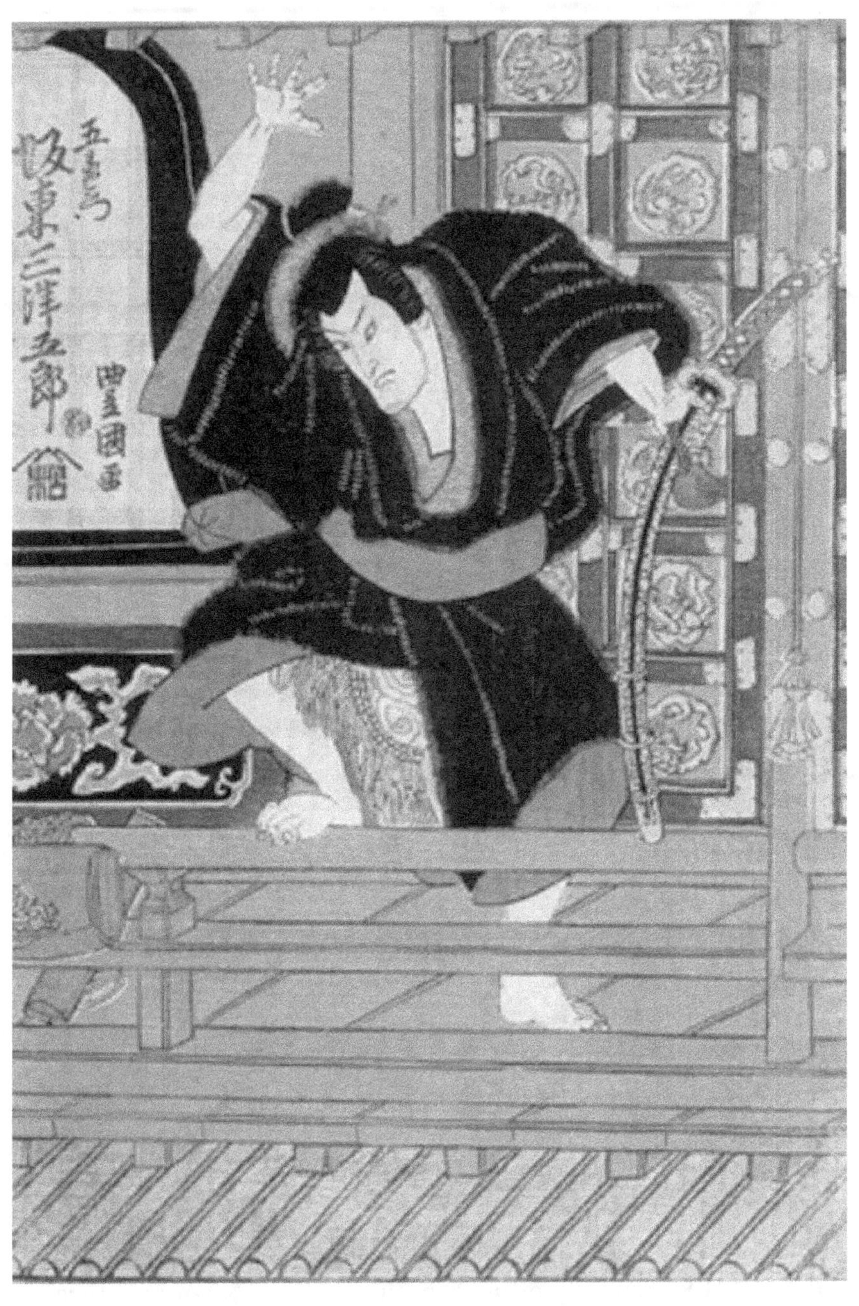

An 1820 woodblock print of Ishikawa Goemon

Recipe: Natto

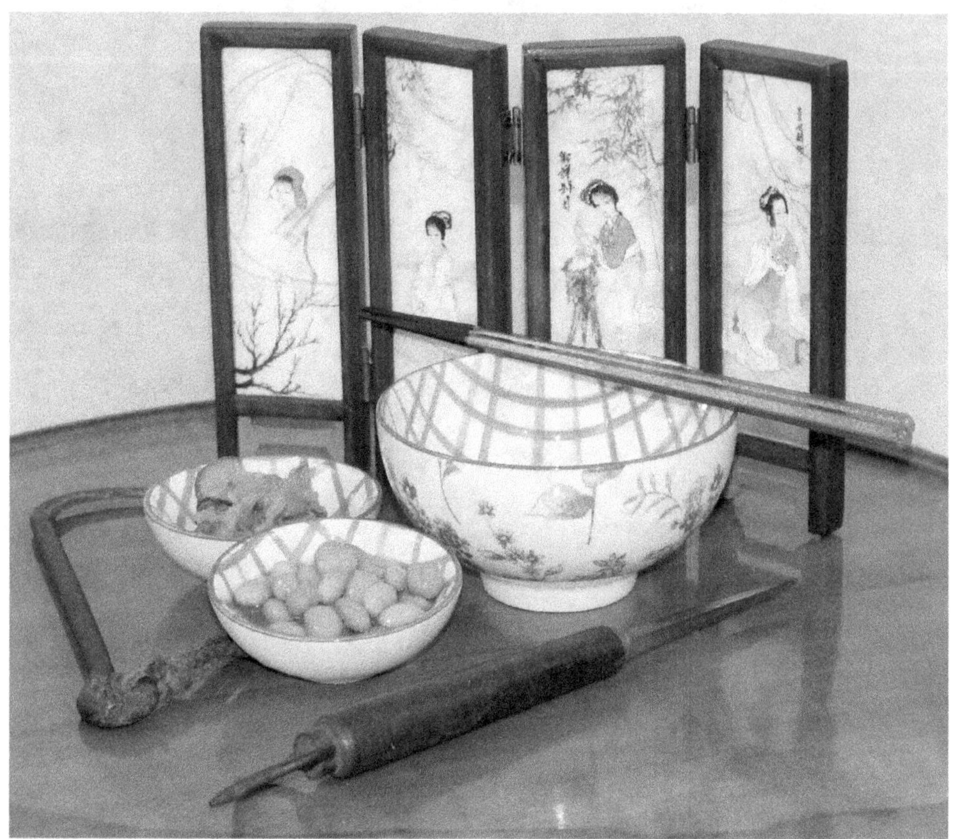

Natto is a fermented soy bean dish that is typically served for breakfast. Natto is known for its health benefits and being a fermented product has a reduced level of complex carbohydrates. Legend tells us that Natto was discovered as a food by the cavalry forces of Minamoto no Yoshiie in 1086 while quelling rebellion in the Mutsu Province of northern Japan. One morning while steaming soy beans Minamoto's encampment was attacked and the beans were quickly packed away. The next day the bags containing the beans were opened and found to be fermented – and Natto was born.

- Soy Beans – 40 parts

- Water – 1 part

- Nattomoto Powder – 1 spoon

The key to making Natto is ensuring everything remains sterile and all utensils must be sterilised before use. The beans are soaked in a large quantity of water for 12 hours and then drained and boiled for a further 9 hours. The Nattomoto Powder is dissolved in two spoons of water and then poured over the warm beans. Spread the beans out in a wide flat covered container and incubate at 37 degrees Celsius or 100 degrees Fahrenheit for a period of 24 hours. Once fermentation is complete allow the beans to cool.

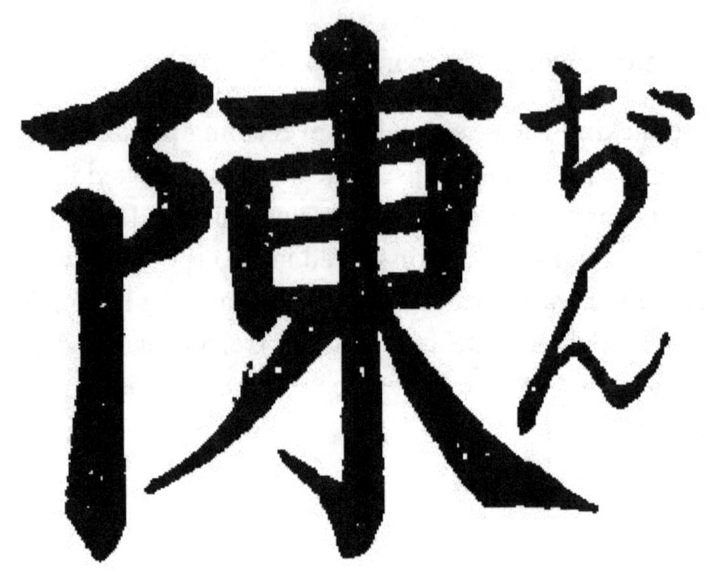

Jin – Awareness – Emotional Intelligence

To perform this *Kuji-in* the practitioner interlocks and crosses over all the fingers and thumbs with the fingers and thumbs remaining on the inside of the hands.

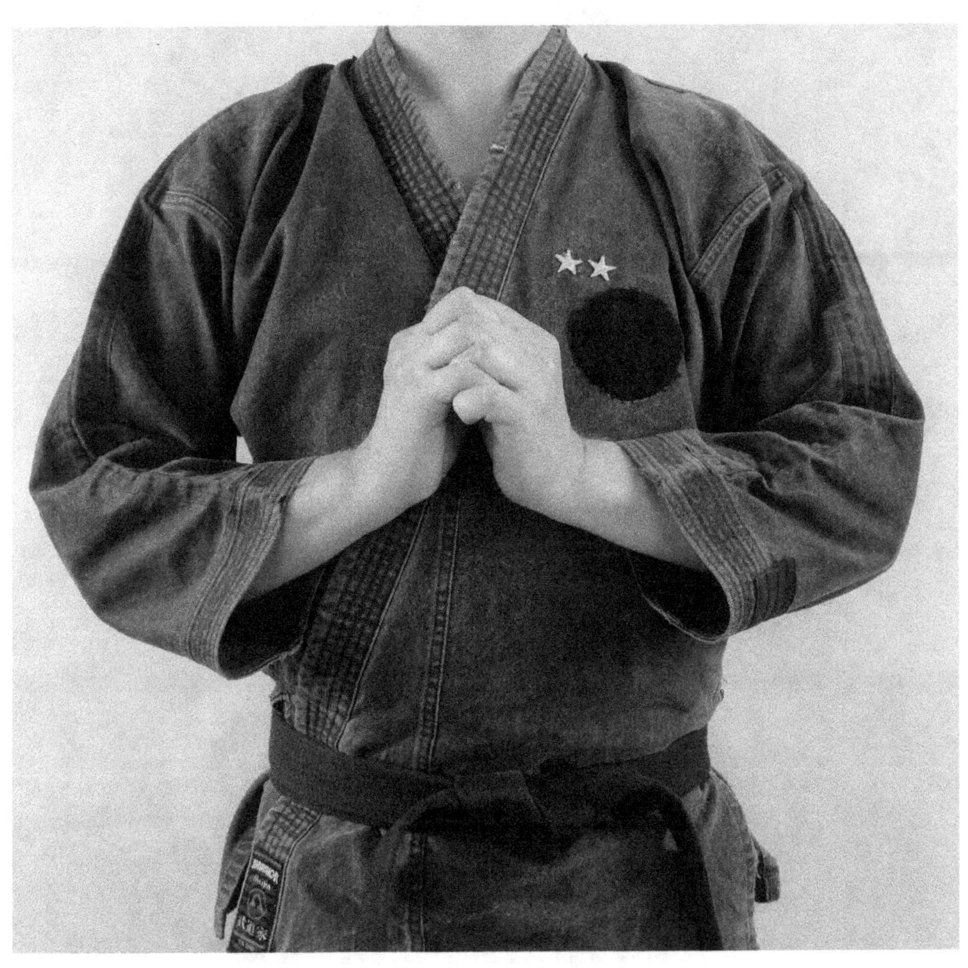

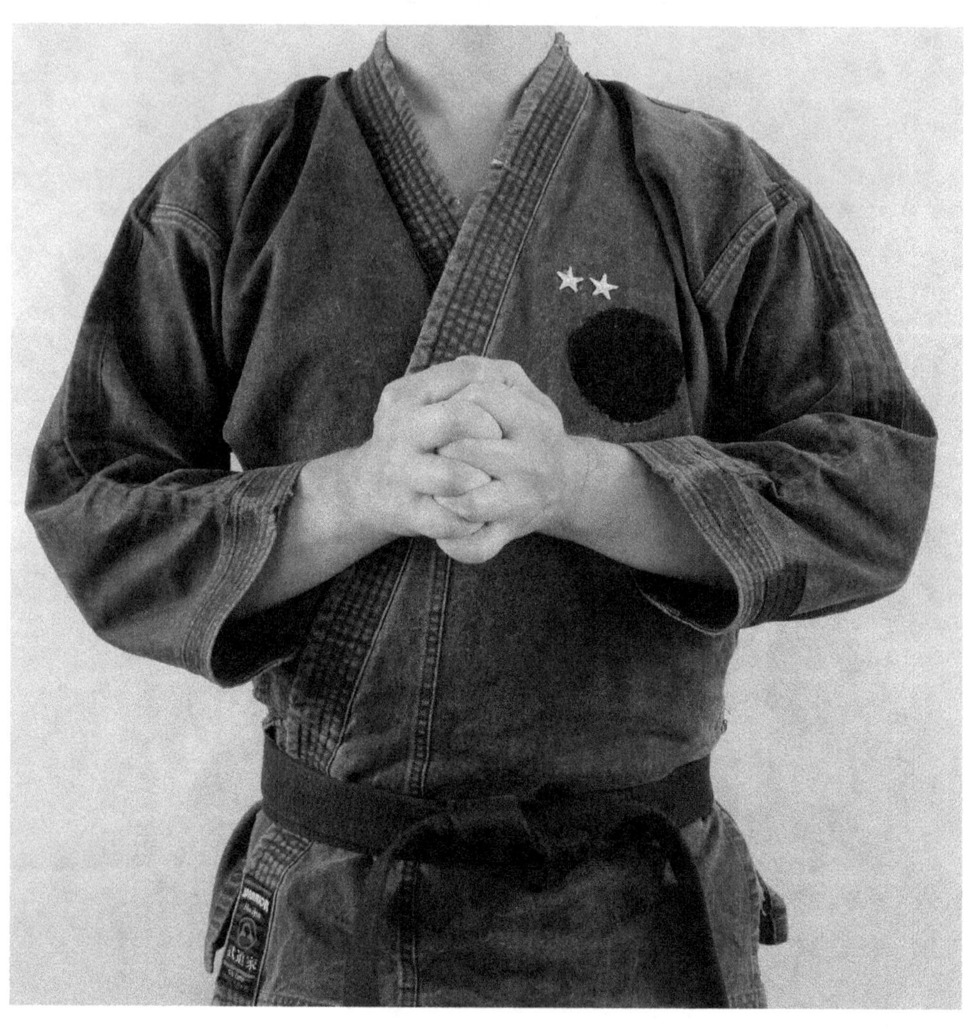

Haiku

The door of thatched hut.
Also changed the owner.
At the Doll's festival.

\- Matsuo Bashō

Legend

Momochi Sandayu is considered to be one of the three greatest *Ninja* of Iga prefecture. Little is specifically known about Momochi Sandayu aside from his exploits in concert with Hattori Hanzo and Fujibayashi Nagato to defend Iga against the forces of Oda Nobunaga during the second Tensho Iga war of 1581.

It has been postulated that Momochi Sandayu and Fujibayashi were the same person and if true is possibly one of the greatest and longest deceptions of all time. It is also known that Momochi Sandayu maintained several households and several wives – also as a deception.

Momochi Sandayu is also known for his principles which were reflected in writings attributed to him:

"Ninjutsu is not something which should be used for personal desires. It is something which should be used when no other choice is available, for the sake of one's country, for the sake of one's lord, or to escape personal danger. If one deliberately uses it for the sake of personal desires, the techniques will indeed fail totally."

Momochi Sandayu is believed to have been killed alongside Fujibayashi Nagato in the penultimate stages of the Tensho Iga war, although, some sources suggest that he escaped to Kii prefecture where he gave up his warrior ways and lived out his life as a farmer.

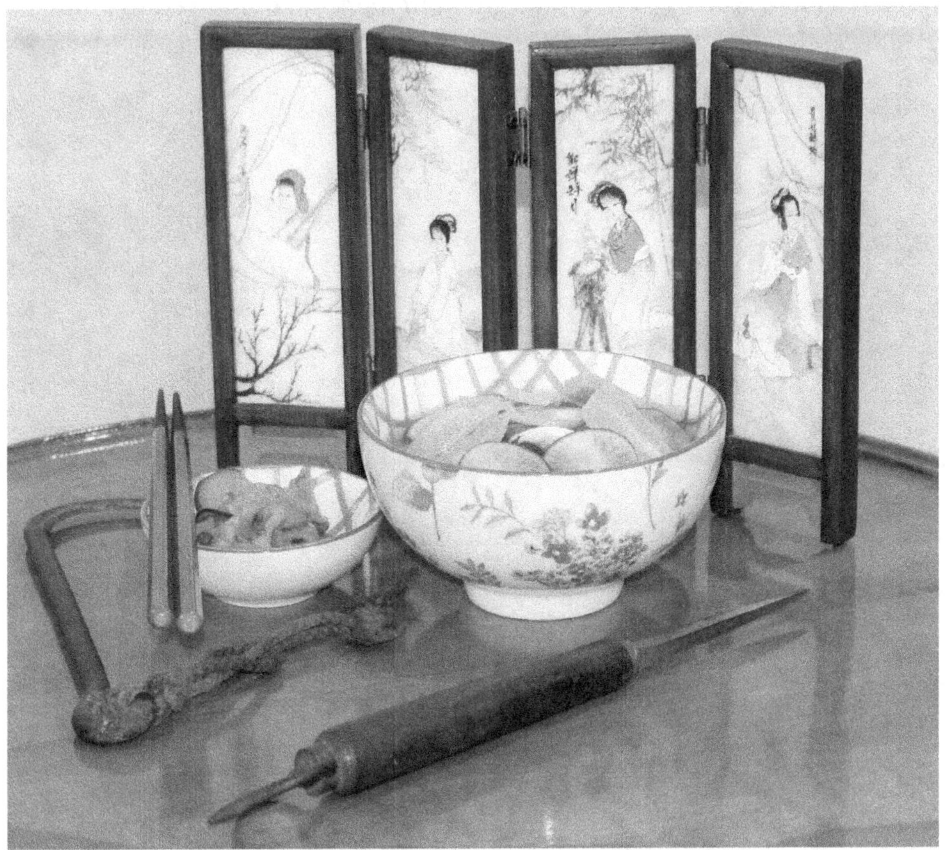

Kamameishi is a traditional rice bowl recipe that changes on the region and season, and seeks to combine the seasonal produce of an area into a heart and filling one bowl meal. Some typical variations include vegetable only (Yasu), eel (Unagi) and the more typical chicken and beef varieties.

- Brown Rice – 5 parts

- Mixed seasonal vegetables (spring onion, carrot, daikom raddish, bamboo shoots, mushroom) – 1 part

- Meat (thin strips of beef, pork, chicken, shimp, eel, clam) – 1 part

- Daishi stock – 1 part

The rice is washed until the water runs clear then allowed to soak for one hour. The rice is then placed in the cooking pot with all the ingredients and water to the top of the ingredients and allowed to simmer for 30 minutes.

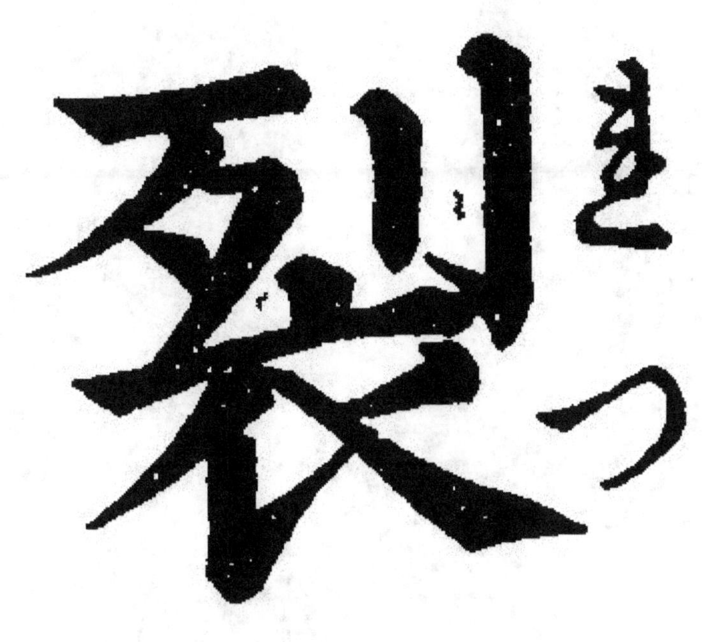

Retsu – Dimension – Omniscience

To perform this *Kuji-in* the practitioner extends the index finger of the left hand, and wraps the fingers of the right hand around it, placing the tip of the index finger of the right hand, against the side of the tip of the index finger on the left hand, and the thumb of the right hand over the tip of the index finger of the left hand.

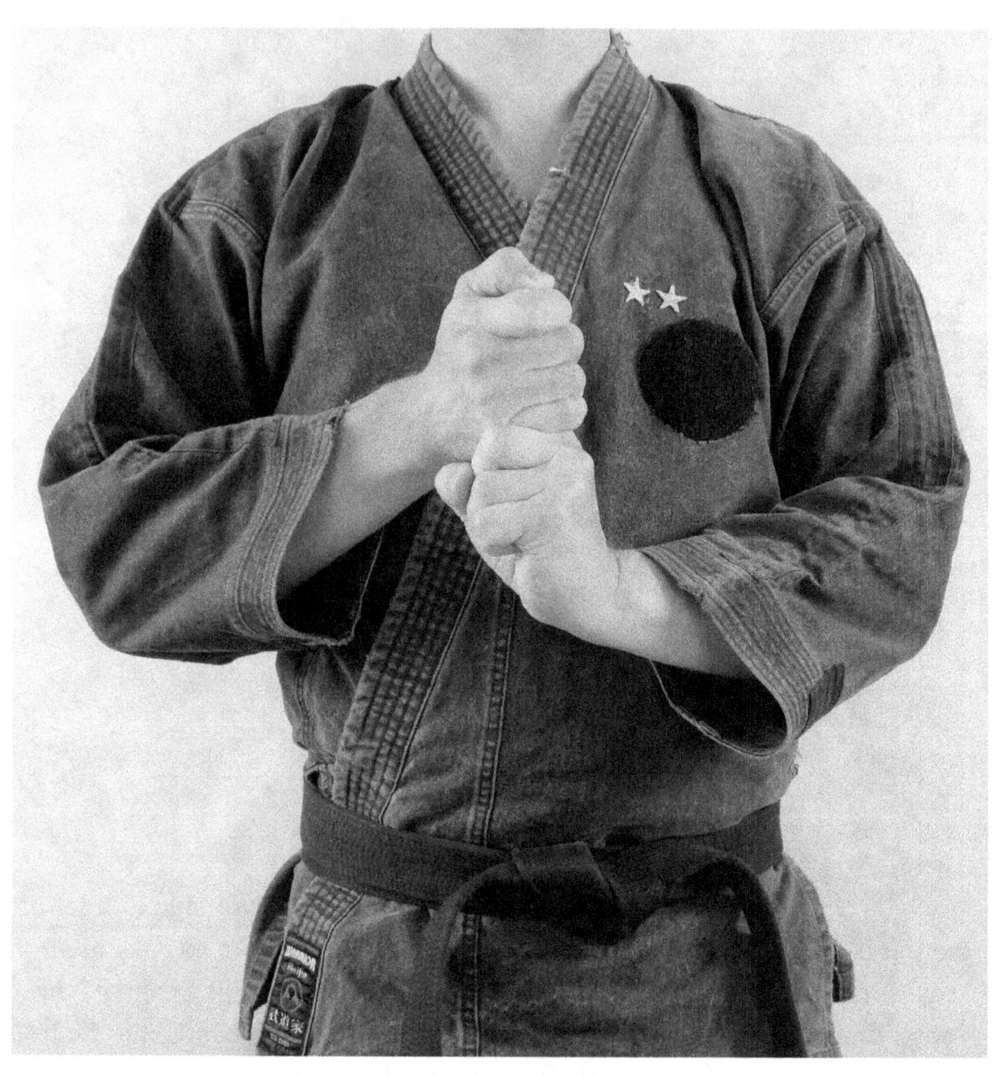

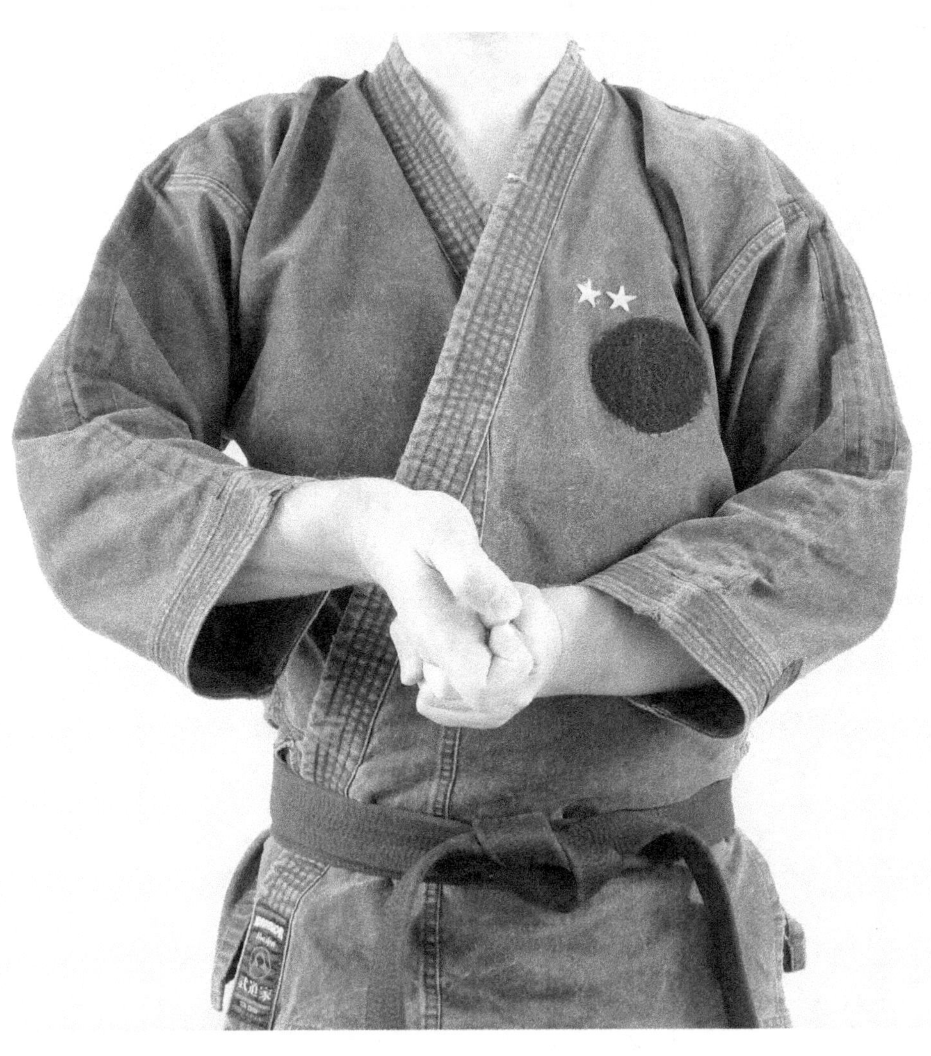

Haiku

An old silent pond...
A frog jumps into the pond,
splash! Silence again.

\- Matsuo Bashō

Legend

Fuma Kotaro was the fifth hereditary leader of the Fuma clan in Kanagawa prefecture and lived from mid to late 1500 and died in 1603. The Fuma clan evolved separately to the more common Koga and Iga clans and specialised in confusion and disruption during battle. The Fuma clan was pledged to the larger and more powerful Odawara clan and performed various services in support of Odawara military campaigns.

In 1580 the Odawara forces gained the attention of Takeda Shingen and Takeda Shingens' son Takeda Katsuyori was sent with a large force to lay siege to the ancestral Odawara home of Hojo castle. The siege lasted some weeks until finally Fuma Kotaro along with some 200 *Ninja* attacked the besieging force by night.

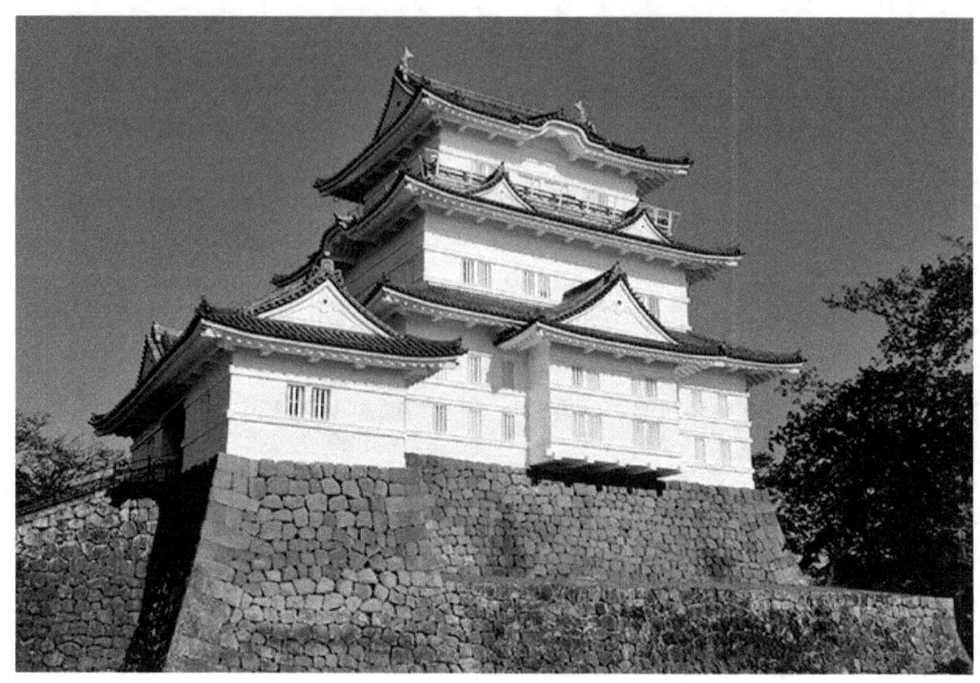

The remains of Hojo Castle today.

Using their tactics of confusion and disruption, Fuma Kotoro convinced different sides of the besieging camp were in fact the enemy, and the entire camp broke into a desperate melee. By dawn the camp was a scene of mass carnage with a significant proportion of the besieging forces wounded or killed, and the siege was lifted.

This was only a delay for the inevitable however. In 1590, Takeda Shingen and Tokugawa Ieyasu attacked and took Hojo castle and ended the Odawara reign. During this time, popular legend told of Fuma Kotaro and Hattori Hanzo battling ultimately with Hattori Hanzo being killed however this is not confirmed. What is known is that Fuma Kotaro met with Kosaka Jinnai in 1596 under a flag of truce however he was betrayed and captured by Tokugawa forces and ultimately beheaded at the order of Tokugawa Ieyasu himself in 1603.

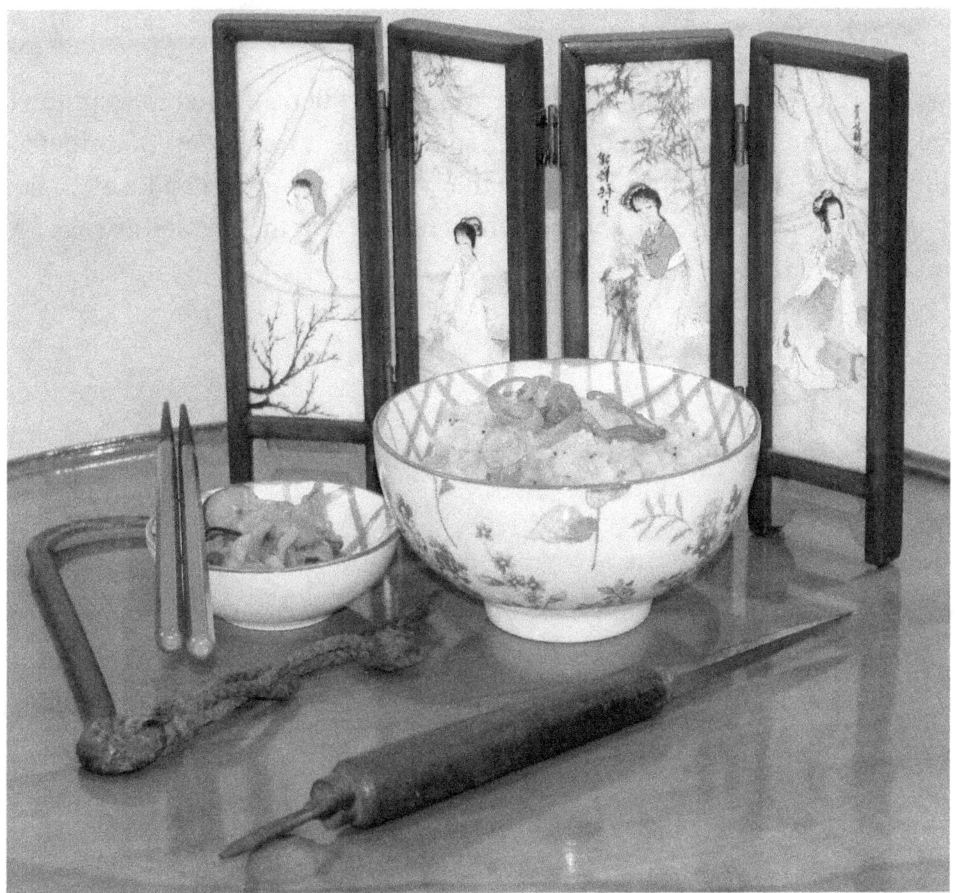

Okayu or Rice Gruel is a high energy food that is dense and sustaining. Rice gruel was transported in bamboo cups and considered to be an expedient food that formed the basis of a diet in the field. Somewhat similar to the use of oats in western diets, rice gruel in its basic form is healthy and sustaining for a body that is subject to physical stress, and also maintains a simplicity which is calming. Anything can be added to rice gruel however do so in very small quantities to maintain a sense of calm subtlety.

- Brown Rice – 10 parts

- Optional Onion, Sesame Seeds, Pickles – 1 part

- Optional Dashi Stock – 1 part

The rice is washed until the water runs clear then allowed to soak for one hour. The rice is then cooked at a medium heat for at least 30 minutes allowing the grains to break up. The thickness of the gruel can be altered by adding water. Any other ingredients are added in the pot at this time and simmered.

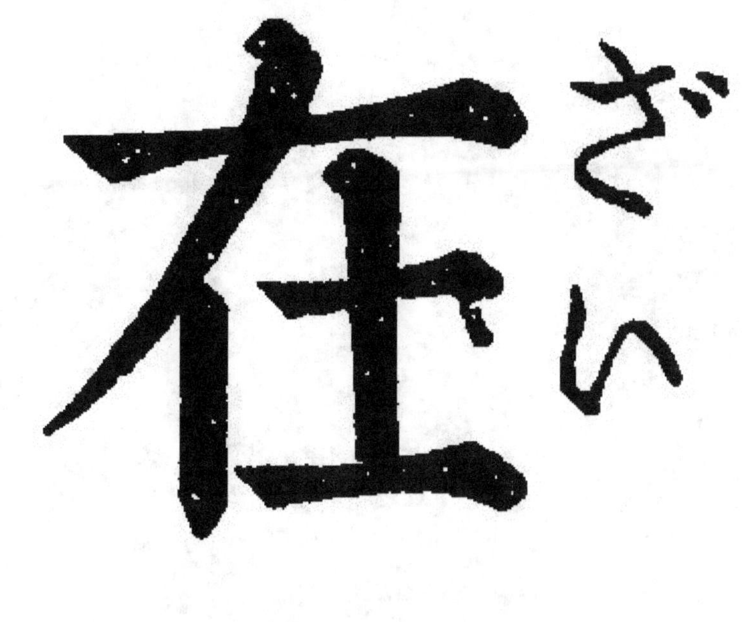

Zai – Creation – Creativity of Though and Resolution

To perform this *Kuji-in* the practitioner extends all the fingers and thumbs and places the tips of the index fingers against each other, and the tips of the thumbs against each other forming a diamond shape.

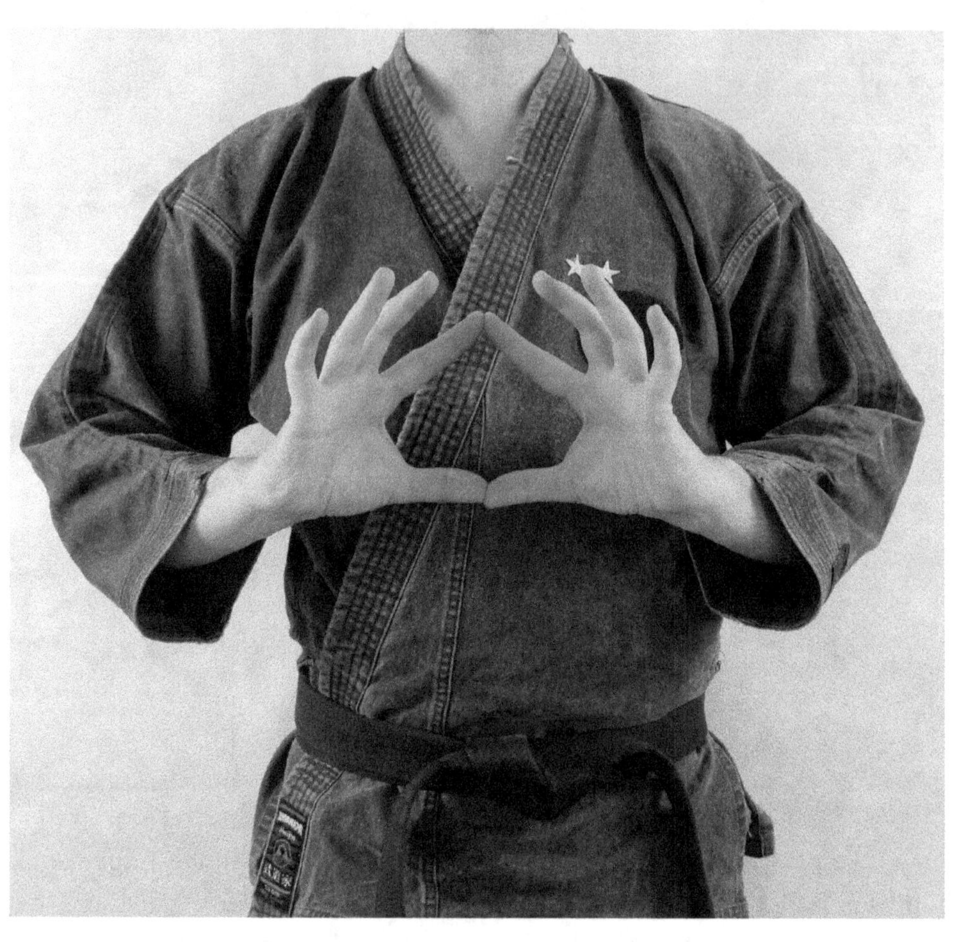

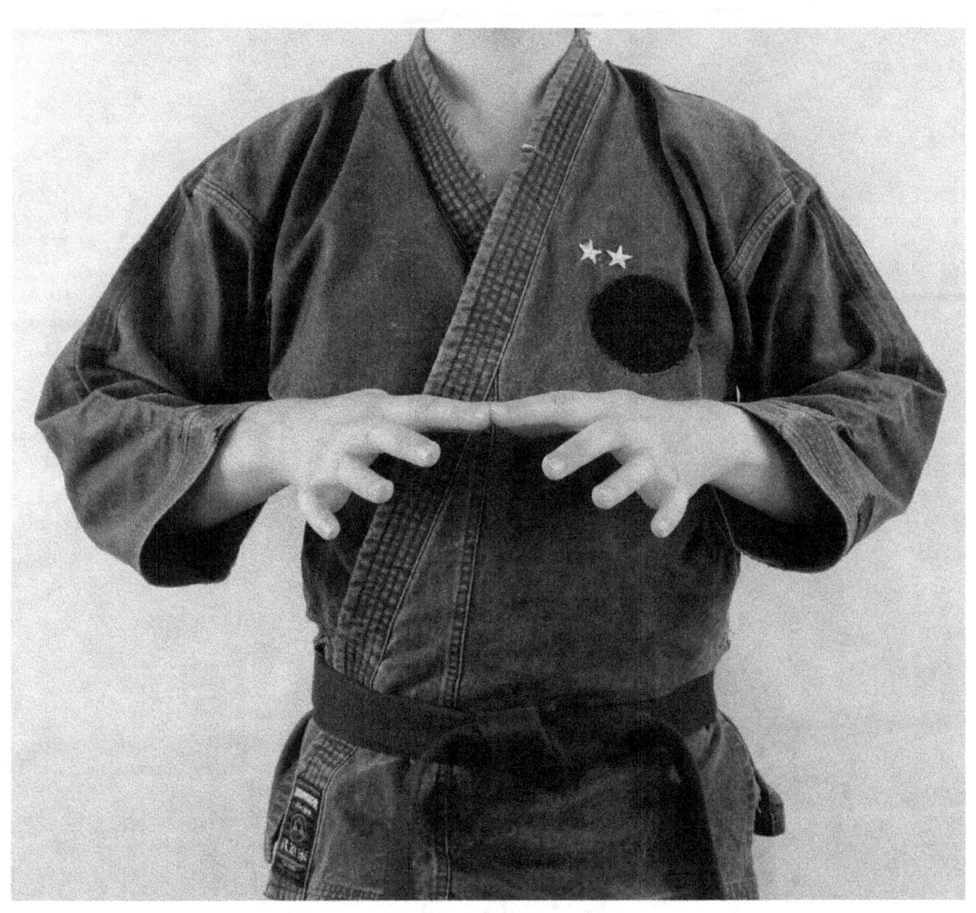

Haiku

My life, -
How much more of it remains?
The night is brief.

- Masaoka Shiki

Legend

Kato Danzo brings the *Ninja* history something of the magic and mysticism that exists behind popular believe of the *Ninja*. Kato Danzo was an illusionist and magician of the Sengoku period and earned his living performing incredible feats. Legend tells us that he was witnessed to have eaten an entire bull in one gulp, caused seeds to immediately sprout and could even fly where he earned the nickname of *Tobi* Kato or flying Kato. It was also believed that Kato Danzo could also hypnotise people around him and cause them to bend to his will or send them to sleep on command.

Kato Danzo gained the attention of Uesugi Kenshin a local *Daimyo* of the Echigo prefecture and was invited into his court as an advisor and spymaster. As a test Kato was tasked with infiltrating the heavily guarded and fortified Sakato castle and stealing a prized *Naginata* or bladed long staff from Uesugi Kenshin's vassal Naoe Kanetsugu. Kato Danzo was successful however the methods that he used are unknown. In fact he was so successful that he was able to steal the *Naginata* and Naoe Kanetsugu's prized servant girl, invoking the wrath of Naoe Kanetsugu.

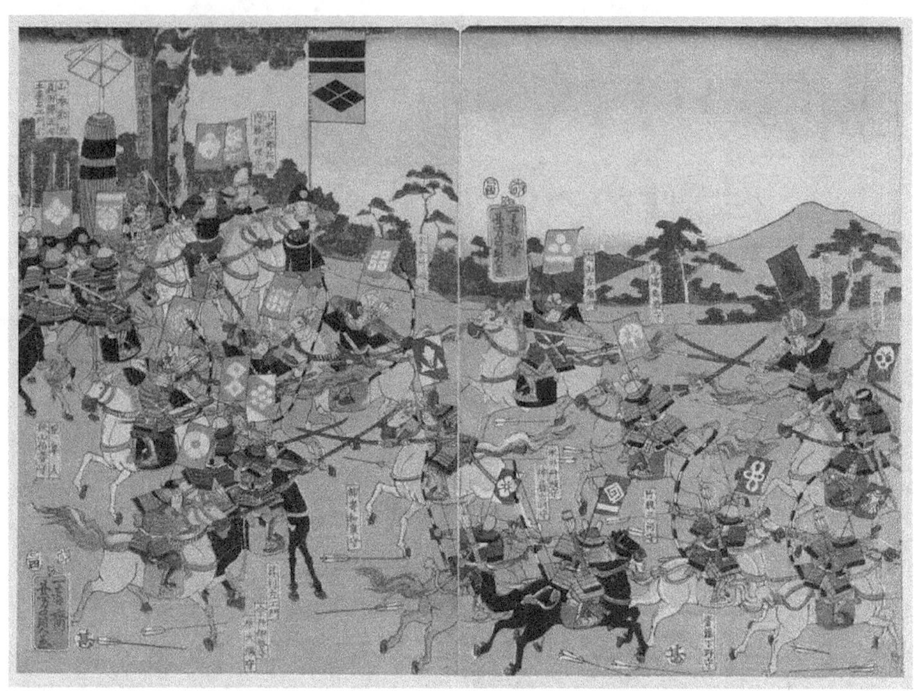

Takeda Shingen and Uesugi Kenshin in battle at Kawanakashima in 1561.

Over time Kato Danzo performed many services for Uesugi Kenshin however he began to fall into disfavour with Uesugi Kenshin possibly due to plotting by the vengeful Naoe Kanetsugu. Kato Danzo took his leave of Uesugi Kenshin and joined with Takeda Shingen – although again due to plotting by Naoe Kanetsugu – was believed by Takeda Shingen to be a spy and was beheaded in 1569.

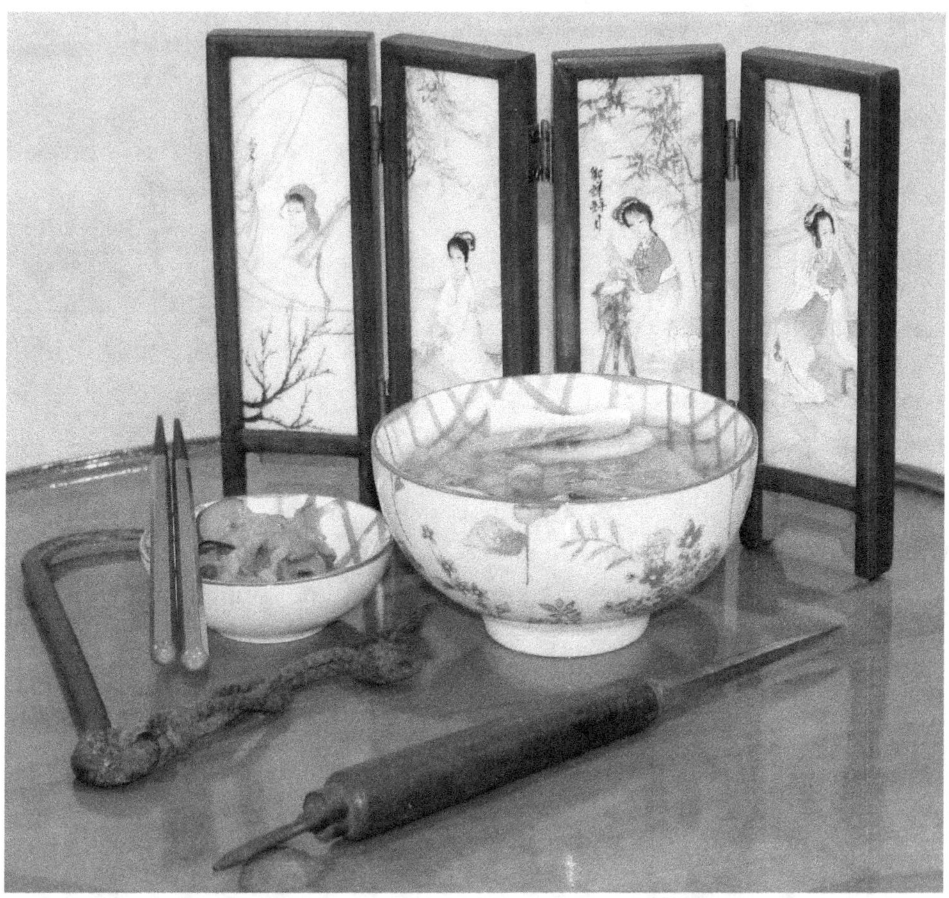

Miyabi or Clear soup is a staple of Japanese cooking and focuses on the use of available vegetables coupled with the fermented spices and seasonings of the region. This dish does not include rice or rice noodles, however it can be combined with both to produce a filling and solid meal. The history of clear soup cannot be traced as it is one of the most fundamental forms of cookery in Japanese culture and while incredibly simple to make, it is both nourishing and adaptable to nearly any situation.

There are a number of variations such as green onion clear soup and some variations use the vegetables to only make stock and then strain out.

- Onion – 1 part

- Carrot – 1 part

- Mushroom – 1 part

- Tofu – 1 part

- Kombu (Dried Kelp) – 1 part

- Water – 10 parts

- Katsuobushi or Bonita Flakes – ½ part

- Sake, Mirin, Soy Sauce – to season

The vegetable ingredients including the tofu are briefly fried over a high heat and set aside. A broth is made using the water and Katsuobushi with small amounts of Sake, Mirin and Soy added to season. The broth is then strained. The vegetables are then added and the soup is simmered for 10 minutes.

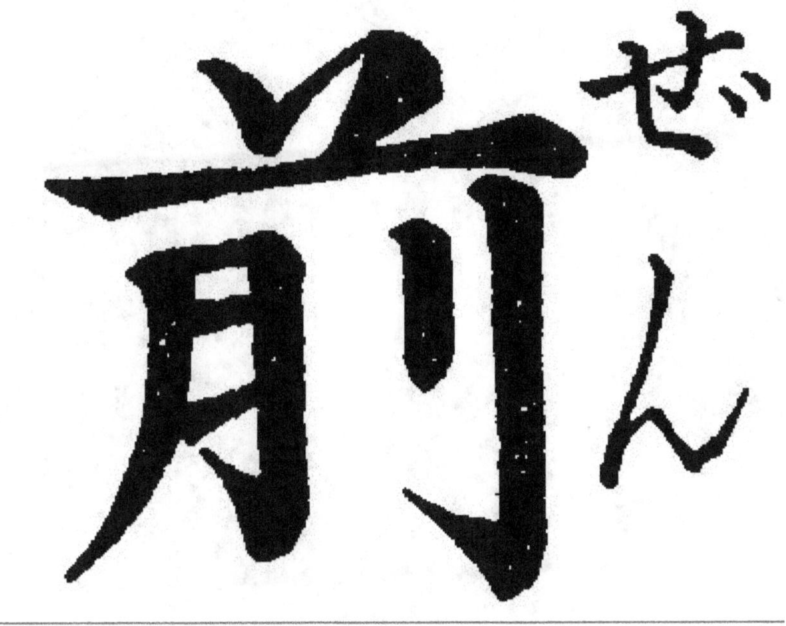

Zen – Absolute – Transcendence

To perform this *Kuji-in* the practitioner makes a crescent shape with each hand and then interlocks both shapes.

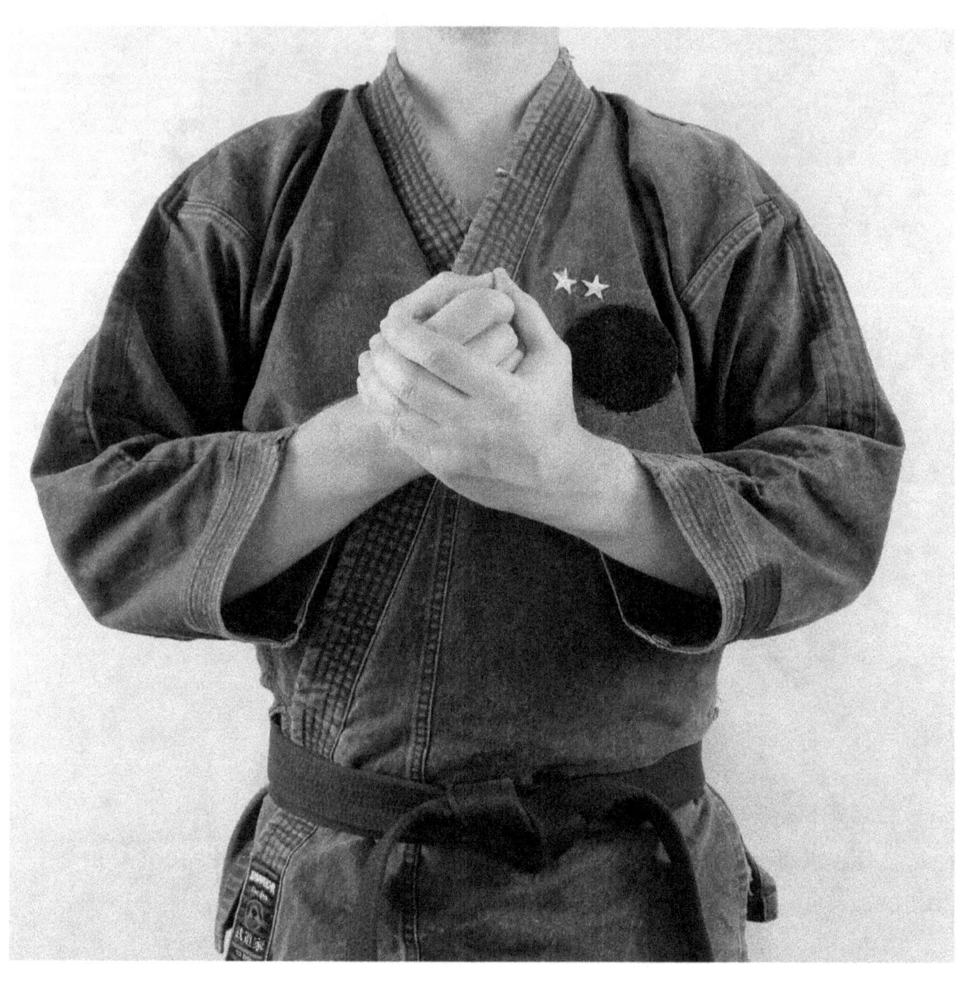

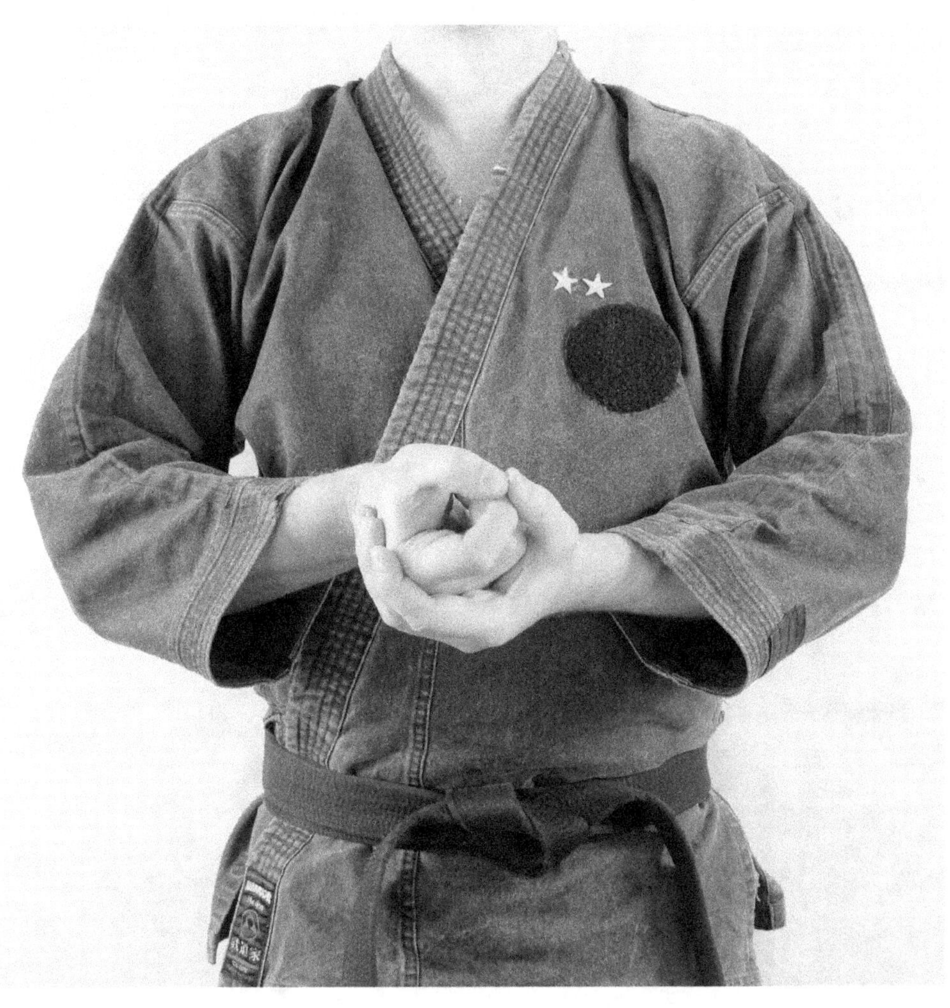

Haiku

Summer grasses
All that remains

The warriors dreams.

- Matsuo Bashō

Legend

Hattori Hanzo is possibly the most well known of *Ninja* to have existed, this isn't to say that he is the greatest *Ninja* of all time, however history has recorded his feats beyond those of others.

Hattori Hanzo was born in 1542 in Iga prefecture to the son of a minor *Samurai* in the service of the Matsudaira clan – a precursor to the Tokugawa clan. Hattori Hanzo studied arms and the military in line with his Iga roots until the age of 16 when he fought his first large scale battle – a night attack on Udo castle and earned his nickname of Oni no Hanzo or Demon Hanzo.

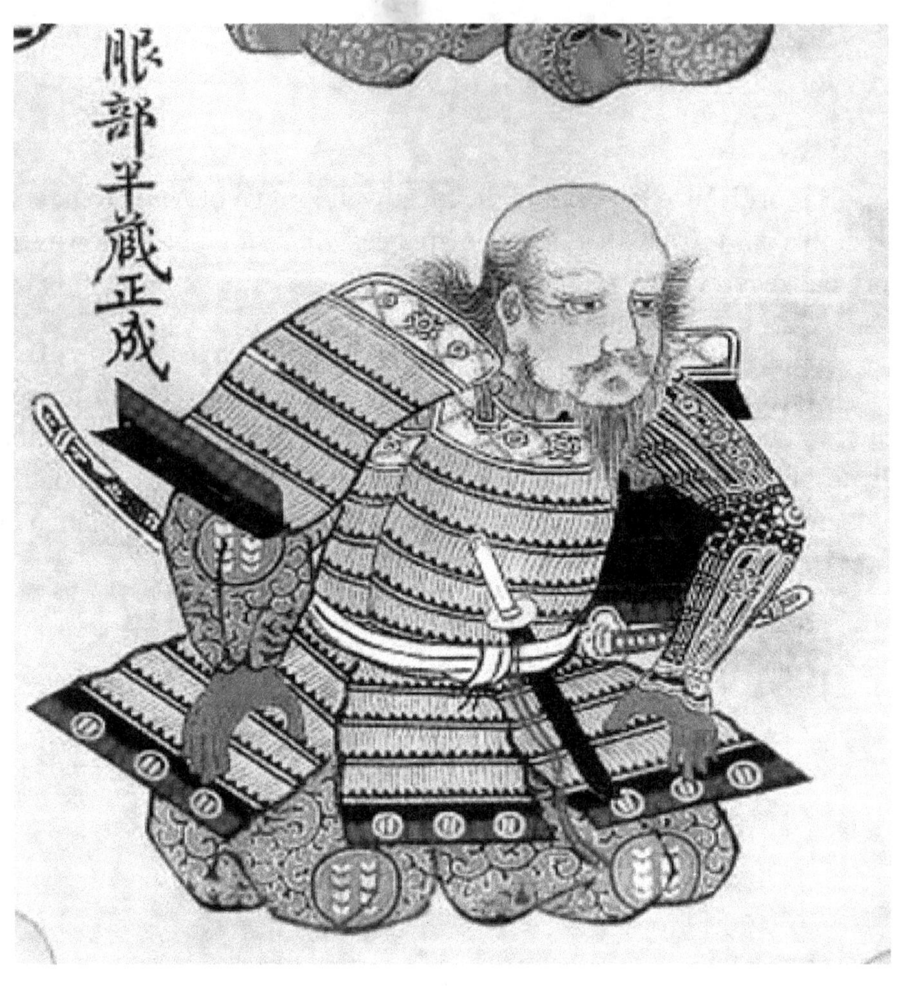

Popular image of Hattori Hanzo circa 1600.

Hattori Hanzo was a master of the spear and a brilliant tactician. Hattori Hanzo was closely linked to Momochi Sandayu and Fujibayashi Nagato in the Iga prefecture and was the co-head of the Iga *Ninja* in the South. Hattori Hanzo played a vital role in the rescue of Tokugawa Ieyasu's and Oda Nobunaga's families during the siege of Kaminogo castle in 1562 and solidified the relationship directly between Hattori Hanzo and Tokugawa Ieyasu.

Hattori Hanzo had a distinguished military career winning the battles of Kakegawa castle in 1569, Anegawa in 1570, Mkatagahara in 1572. When Tokugawa Ieyasu's son was accused of treason and ordered to commit *Seppuku* or ritual suicide, Hattori Hanzo was asked by Tokugawa Ieyasu to act as second and behead his son, to which Hattori Hanzo refused to draw the blood of his lord, bringing Tokugawa Ieyasu again to realise the strength of loyalty that Hattori Hanzo maintained to the Tokugawa clan. Tokugawa Ieyasu upon hearing this commented that 'even a demon can shed tears'.

Hattori Hanzo is perhaps best known for his fighting withdrawal across Mikawa prefecture in 1582 where he and a group of both Iga and Koga *Ninja* protected and guarded Tokugawa Ieyasu, the *Shogun* designate, from constant and overwhelming attack as he returned to Edo castle to take up his post. As a result of this heroic action, the Iga and Koga *Ninja* were made the palace guard at Edo castle and became the special agents of the Tokugawa *Shogunate*.

It is believed that Hattori Hanzo died at age 55 in 1596, however in line with his family tradition, his son took the name Hattori Hanzo, adding to the belief that Hattori Hanzo was immortal.

Today, the Imperial Palace in Tokyo maintains the Hanzomon or Hanzo's Gate and Hatori Hanzo's spear, helmet and armour rest alongside his remains in the Sainen-Ji Temple in Yotsuya, Tokyo.

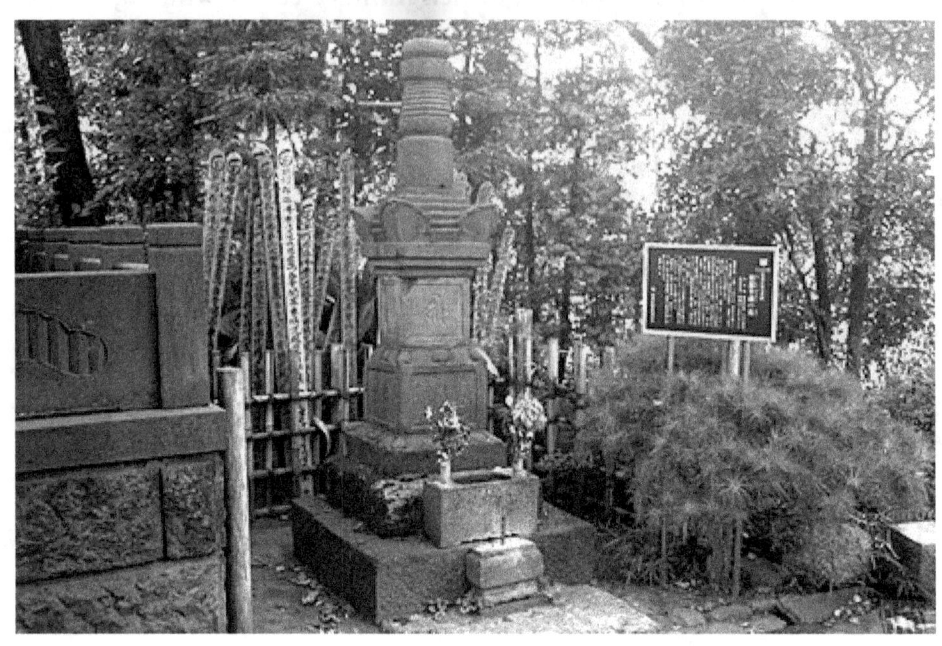

The grave of Hattori Hanzo today.

Recipe: Motsunabe

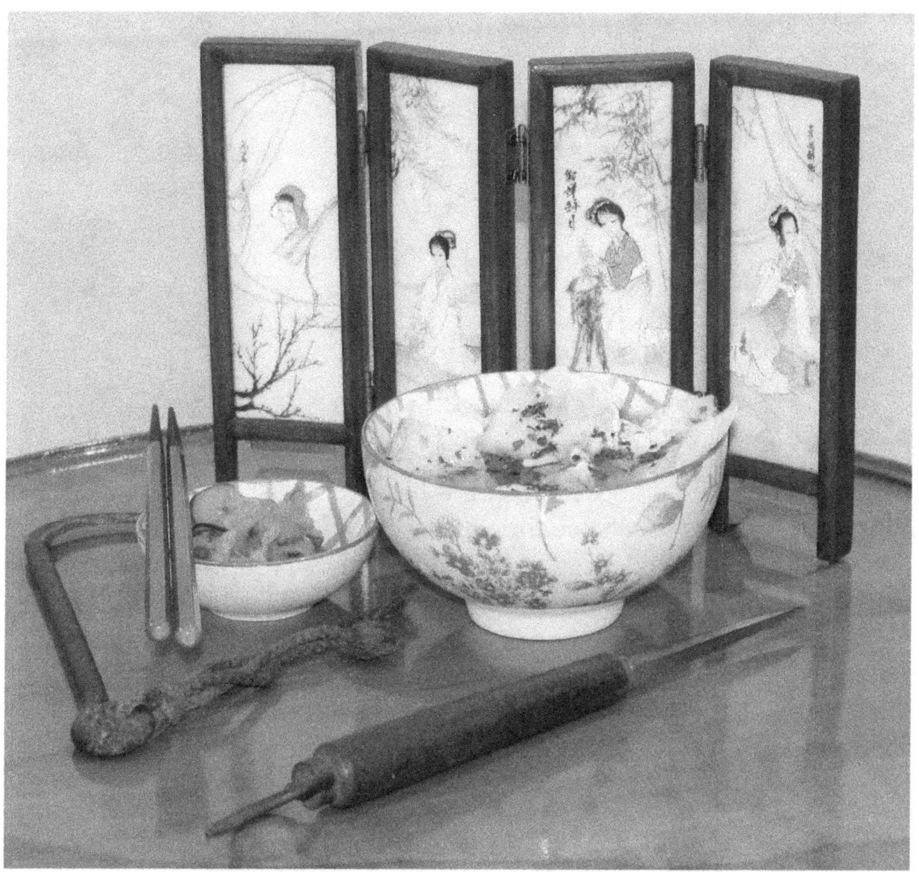

Motsunabe or beef guts stew is a dish that has a checkered history. Focusing on a way to use the offal parts of beef and pork that spoiled quickly, this was a dish that could be cooked and eaten immediately while the more favourable parts of the beast were reserved for sale or preserving. While this dish can be made using primarily intestine, any offal can be substituted, or for that matter, any cut of meat.

- Intestine, Offal or any kind of meat – 1 part

- Cabbage – 1 part

- Bean Sprouts – 1 part

- Chives – 1 part

- Water – 4 parts

- Dashi stock – ½ part

- Garlic – to season

- Chili – to season

- Soy Sauce – to season

- Sweet Sake – to season

- Ginger – to season

If offal of any kind is used ensure it has been washed and blanched in boiling water before use. Slice the vegetables and meat into medium size pieces that are thin. Mix the water, Dashi, Garlic, Chili, Soy, Sake and Ginger and bring to a slow boil over a medium heat. Add the meat and cook for five minutes. Add the vegetables and remove from the heat and allow the Motsunabe to steep for ten minutes. It may require adding further Soy, Sake, Ginger and Dashi to taste prior to eating.

Closing Notes

The pursuit of any meaningful goal is an exercise in perseverance and it is through this challenge that the Human mind experiences the joy of accomplishment. Although there are no 'silver bullets' for success or miracle solutions to problems, if there were, they would rob us of this experience of challenge and triumph and rob us also of the joy of daily living.

The Ninja diet tells us that the joy is in the moment and that we must cherish every moment and understand that individual events are neither good nor bad as we are so inclined to constantly categorise our every moment of existence.

In closing, the sense of accomplishment that we feel for having overcome a challenge is directly linked to the magnitude of the challenge and so in our daily lives it is important to sense the accomplishment in all tasks and in all ways. It is this building block that will give us the fortitude and perseverance to succeed.

About the Author

David Watson is a student of *Kobudo* or 'old' Japanese martial arts. David has attained a 7th Dan black belt in a traditional battlefield art and regularly travels to Japan to study and learn about the culture, history and essence of martial arts, and to learn from the grand master of his school.

David brings this book to us to pass on some the knowledge and life lessons that he has learned during his studies and travels and asks us to consider a different way of thinking in the pursuit of our goals.

David's intention is that we should all be able to incorporate aspects of this book into our daily lives and develop a sense of calm and to be at peace in a world that becomes more frantic with each passing day.

-Bufu Ikkan

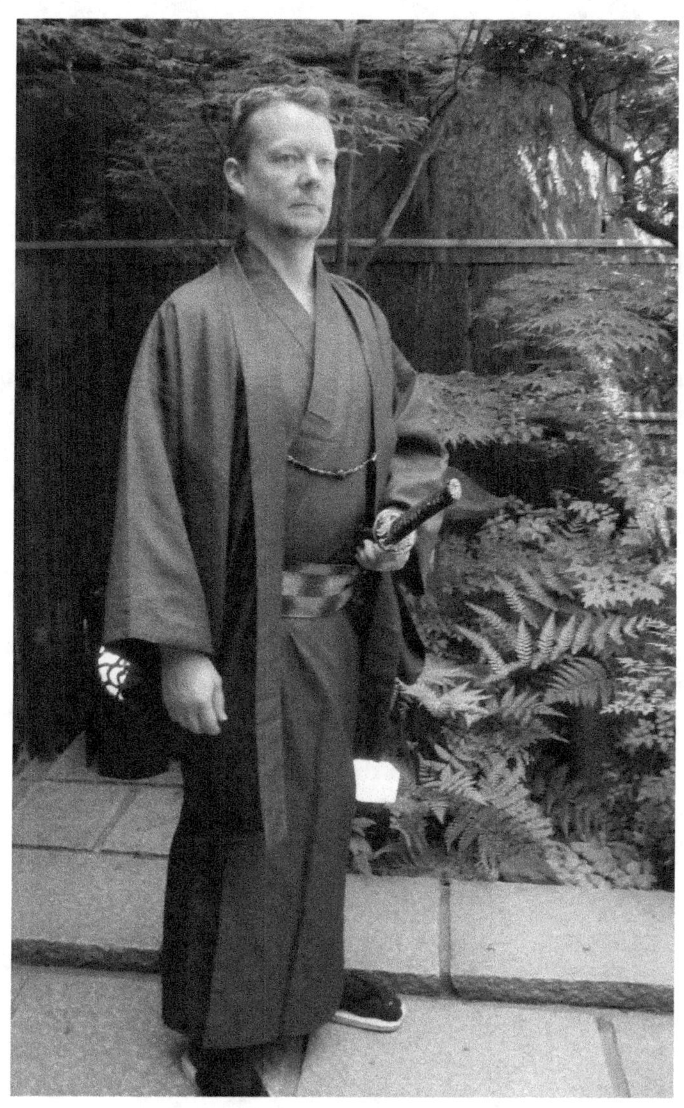

The author recently in Kyoto.